THE
ALKALINE DIET

Mark Blair

Introduction

Thank you for purchasing this informative book! I am sure you will like every bit of it.

Before we begin, tell me something-

Are you suffering from any medical problems like indigestion, stomach bloating, headaches or the more serious ones like arthritis, heart disease, diabetes, osteoporosis or even cancer- or just feeling like your health is not like before?

Do you usually feel groggy, sluggish, tired, too heavy or lethargic during the day even after having a good night's sleep? Do you struggle with nagging cravings which are clearly sabotaging your efforts to live a healthy life?

Are you concerned with your weight gain and are having a problem losing fat (you've probably even tried dieting, working out and fasting) but the only thing you're losing is your mind (and patience)? Are you usually stressed out (sometimes for no good reason) and worried that your condition may worsen and probably get you diagnosed with depression or ulcers?

If you answered 'yes' to at least ONE of the questions above, then you need this book to learn why you're not okay, and why you need the alkaline diet to improve your situation. The alkaline diet is not making conversations all over the world, changing lives and saving lives for no reason- and don't forget that all the symptoms I've highlighted above are just the tip of the iceberg, as there are thousands more; these symptoms underlie a bigger problem known as body acidity which everyone who's not on the alkaline diet has.

You just need to address yours as soon as you can. Even if you are not suffering from any of the symptoms above, you want to feel younger, more energetic, stay away from illnesses and feel happier and healthier. I am giving you that missing piece that you need to lead a completely fulfilled life.

This book is therefore everything you need to know about the alkaline diet and how to incorporate it in your life.

You'll learn the following and more:

- The role of pH in the body, including what happens when the pH is low in your body (when you're acidic)

- Why you need to do something about your body pH to create a less acidic environment

- How to alkalize your body with common foods and drinks

- How to control your body weight (and lose weight)

- All you need to know about some of the most important medicinal herbs and the best ways to prepare them in addition to their main uses.

- And much more

Welcome to your alkaline diet guide!

Thanks again for purchasing this book. I hope you enjoy it!

About Author

For a long time, Mark has always been passionate about healthy living. This perhaps explains why he opted to pursue a degree in Pharmacy then went on to do his MSc in Transfusion and Transplantation Sciences at the University of Bristol, UK.

Despite his academic qualifications, he still strongly believes that the body's internal healing mechanisms are the best solution for healthy living. He also strongly believes that diet is the greatest determinant of how our lives turn out, especially regarding our health.

That's why he doesn't shy away from recommending certain diets to his friends and colleagues, as he understands that when you 'hack' the diet part, you are well on your way to living a healthier, happier and more fulfilling life.

This book is top on the list of Mark's recommendations, as it features a way of eating that Mark has seen work in the lives of countless people in his line of work.

Table of Contents

The Meaning And Basics Of The Alkaline Diet

Health is a state of total harmony of body, mind and spirit. This harmony is achieved best when you feed yourself well as every bit of food you take affects your health either positively or negatively (there's no middle ground). The foods you eat are the building blocks for your cells, tissues and organs and they definitely have the ability to increase or reduce your waistline, make your skin and hair look good or messed up, make you feel groggy or energetic and lively or even increase or reduce your chances of developing all kinds of diseases and conditions. The alkaline diet is the best approach you can take to influence how you feel and look- through food- without feeling like you're trying too hard.

Also known as the acid-alkaline diet as well as the alkaline ash diet, the alkaline diet is a style of eating that centers heavily on vegetables and fruits instead of meats and grains, which most of us are used to. It's based on the premise that eating certain foods positively influences the acid-base homeostasis or equilibrium, which is essential when it comes to healing and maintaining a good body health.

Advocates of the alkaline diet assert that everyday health problems are caused by certain foods which offset this balance by making the body more acidic. The alkaline diet is basically alkaline forming, and is generally high in alkaline minerals and compounds such as magnesium, bicarbonate and potassium.

The Alkaline Diet And pH

The pH (potential of hydrogen) is the measure of alkalinity or acidity of substances that are soluble in water. On a pH scale, value 0 represents "most acidic" and value 14 represents "most alkaline". A pH of 7 is neutral.

The purpose of adopting an alkaline diet is to assist your body maintain a normal pH range (mentioned above) and counter the effects of foods you've been eating that have been lowering the pH. In any case- as you will learn shortly, what you eat influences the level of compensation the body has to do. Foods such as red meat, dairy products, alcohol, processed foods, alcohol and sugars are acid forming; they increase the toxin load in the body and cause metabolic acidosis (they raise acidity when they are processed for energy).

If you are ardent about reducing your risk of chronic illness, you have to correct your pH levels. As I am going to explain in detail, high acid levels in the body increase the risk of developing degenerative diseases, diabetes, hypertension and so many other diseases and conditions that generally reduce your lifespan. Unless you want to die younger than you should, then adopting the alkaline diet is extremely important.

Acidity and degenerative diseases

According to a study conducted back in 2012 that was published in The Journal of Environmental and Public Health (Schwalfenberg, 2012), consuming an alkaline diet can reduce the chances of mortality caused by chronic disease. According to this study's findings, chronic acidosis causes bone disease because it contributes to decreased bone density.

What happens is that the presence of high acidity makes the body pull calcium (which is an essential alkaline mineral in the body) from the bones to try and restore the right body pH. As the acidity in the body increases, the body uses the calcium in the bones until the calcium is in very low levels. As you would expect, this reduces the density of the bones and eventually gives rise to bone disease.

This study also discovered that body acidosis contributes to muscle loss as we age, which increases the risk of falling and having fractures. This three-year-long study published in the US National Library of Medicine (Dawson-Hughes, 2008) found that consuming alkaline forming vegetables and fruits (which are particularly rich in potassium) assists in reducing the acid load in the bodies of older persons and preserving their muscle mass. You need to note that when your skeletal muscles break down, you are at a greater risk of experiencing lung disease, renal failure sepsis, chronic obstructive lung disease, sepsis and trauma.

Acidity and insulin resistance

According to research (McCarty), an acidic diet that particularly comprises animal protein and starchy foods can negatively affect the release of insulin in the body, which may affect the body in many ways, including increasing the risk of becoming diabetic.

Insulin is a hormone that is responsible for maintaining balance in blood sugar levels in the body, and managing fat storage. It is produced to help carry glucose (obtained from food) into the cells to be used as energy (it works by signaling the insulin receptors in cells to open up so as to take up glucose). It also facilitates the storage of excess glucose as glycogen molecule in the liver as well as fat to be used as energy later when the need arises. Therefore, apart from maintaining a balance in the blood sugar levels, insulin also has a role to play in the metabolism of fat.

Note that as you consume insulin-spiking foods or high glycemic index foods (which are usually discouraged in the alkaline diet) such as processed foods and refined sugars, the body requires more and more insulin to maintain the stability of blood sugar levels.

As you'd expect, this can cause lots of fat accumulation over time and if the diet remains the same, this can continue until your body stops responding to insulin. In this case, we say that you've started developing insulin resistance. When this takes place (the insulin stops working properly), it's highly unlikely that you'll be able to shake off the belly fat even with physical exercises.

Put differently, insulin is like a key that unlocks the cells for sugar to get in; this in turn enables your body to use the food you are eating. Nonetheless, factors such as excess and unhealthy food can cause this 'key' to get stuck, or have a problem getting into the lock. If it is lucky enough to get in, turning the 'lock' can also become a problem, thus the term 'resistant'. If your body becomes resistant to insulin, you cannot be able to effectively utilize the food you take in, and that can cause constant fatigue and loss of focus since your body is not getting enough energy, and your cravings for more insulin-spiking foods will increase as your body seeks energy.

Indeed, sugar is a key culprit in weight gain, and this fact is supported by studies including this one by (Stanhope, 2016)

We'll discuss more on sugar shortly.

Generally speaking, you'll start experiencing the following symptoms-apart from an increase in belly fat:

- Fatigue after meals

- Blood sugar swings or hypoglycemia

- Problems with blood clotting

- Sugar cravings

- High triglycerides

- Low sex drive

While the obvious solution to this would be to reduce your intake of processed foods and other high-glycemic index foods such as cakes, white rice, pasta and other simple carbohydrates, which create acidity in the body and replace them with more whole foods, the alkaline diet gives you a better option that has been proven to work.

The studies below are some of the many that conclude that the alkaline diet is made up of the right foods to reduce insulin resistance and protect against the development of diseases and conditions that arise in consequence, such as type 2 diabetes.

(Williams, 2016)

(Williams R. S.-B., 2016)

Besides increasing insulin sensitivity, alkaline diet foods, which are low in animal protein have been seen to promote the breakdown of fats in the body through another hormone known as glucagon.

This study by (Scott, 2018), which sought to find a solution to type II diabetes found glucagon an important factor in supporting weight loss because it reduces food intake and increases energy expenditure in the body, which is vital in reducing obesity.

The role of cortisol

When you take acidic foods for an extended period of time, one of the things that could result is an increase in the levels of a hormone known as cortisol. When in controlled levels in the bloodstream, cortisol can be beneficial, as it can lead to a better memory function, quick bursts of energy (for survival reasons), healthy immunity and so forth.

However, when the hormone remains elevated in the blood for long periods of time, it can lead to the following:

- Impaired cognitive function

- Reduced bone density

- Suppressed thyroid performance

- Hyperglycemia and other forms of blood sugar imbalances

- Increased blood pressure

- Reduced muscle tissue

- Reduced inflammatory responses in the body and lowered immunity

What's worse; this hormone also causes insulin resistance. In this case, it sort of acts like what scientists call an 'insular-hormone', which means that it is able to inhibit the signaling of insulin in peripheral tissues like adipocytes (fat cells) and the skeletal muscles.

This study by (PEDERSEN, 1996) will help you to learn more.

Actually, scientists have realized that visceral fat cell receptors are usually a lot more responsive to cortisol than the subcutaneous fat (also known as the active fat, visceral fat is the type of fat that is deposited around your body organs. Subcutaneous fat is the type that lies directly beneath your skin).

This further highlights a possible connection between increased cortisol and the lack of a glucose balance or homeostasis in the blood because a lack of proper functioning of the fat cells (or adipocytes) is usually significant in the development of insulin resistance. These studies provide more details on the exact mechanisms:

(Rebuffé-Scrive, 1990)

(Maurizi, 2018)

According to studies, the secretion of cortisol is stimulated by low pH (acidity) as such an environment helps in clearing excess hydrogen ions:

(Hamm, 1999)

(Bailey, 2000)

In this regard, Buehlmeier et al (Buehlmeier, 2016), observed an overall reduction in the secretion of cortisol when alkali supplementation was introduced in the study (they essentially pooled results from randomized trials to come up with their results).

Given the nature of cortisol, this study by (ANNA CHALLA, 1993) also found that increasing its amount in the body as a result of metabolic acidosis (which comes from the metabolism of acidic foods) makes insulin sensitivity worse:

More sugar problems

We've already seen that sugar can convert to belly fat, and lead to obesity, among other problems. To make matters worse, studies have also found that sugar affects the brain's health significantly.

For instance, this study (Despa, 2013) found that sugar causes a buildup of a type of protein that is produced in the bone marrow known as amyloid protein, which is toxic and linked with dementia:

To support this study, this report by Stanhope (Stanhope, 2016) showed that older adults who were used to consuming a lot of sugar and simple carbohydrates were more likely to develop dementia compared to their counterparts who generally consumed lower levels of such foods.

The fact is that we are consuming more sugar than ever before. From 1977 to 1978 and 1994 to 1996, the average daily consumption of added sugars by the average American increased by 35% (from 235 to 318 calories). This huge increase is mainly attributed to soft drinks, which is the one of the highest source of calories.

Currently, more than 10 percent of the daily calories of Americans come from sugar-sweetened beverages, foods that contain grains as well as fruit juice which is mainly made up of sugar. (Vos, 2008)

Lastly, according to research (Schwalfenberg, 2012), the alkaline state is the best for your body's optimal health, and most cells and tissues maintain an alkaline pH balance. Sugar causes an imbalance to the pH and creates acidity, putting you at risk of even more problems such as kidney stones, oxidative stress and chronic inflammation. Besides what we've already discussed, excess sugar also creates an imbalance in potassium and sodium in the body, thus encouraging to a more acidic environment.

When you combine that with loss of calcium in the body and the reduction of sodium bicarbonate (which is usually referred to as a key buffer in the body), you've got yourself the perfect combo for metabolic acidosis:

Acidity and cancer

Acidity is a well-known factor that is linked with cancer. When you have low pH between the body cells, you are at risk of developing cancerous cells because that's an ideal environment for their growth and this has been studied and shown to be true: (Robey, 2012)

When you have chronic acidosis, which indicates that you are consuming an overly acidic diet, you may get hyperinsulinema, a condition that is characterized by high levels of circulating insulin. This condition is linked with the pancreatic and colorectal cancers as well as breast cancer, kidney cancer and endometrial cancer. The study above has more details on this.

We have always known that cancer usually evolves from genetic factors or their changes in the normal cell, but today, we'll talk about how "alkaline ash" and mitochondrial dysfunction in the context of metabolic acidosis can give rise to cancer.

1: Alkaline ash

Our bodies have been designed to maintain alkaline reserves that are used to sort of neutralize acids when they increase within the body but most of us have already depleted our reserves. When the buffering/neutralizing system is overrun by acidity, the body starts dumping the excess acids into the tissues. As more and more acid accumulates, the tissues start deteriorating and the acid wastes oxidize or 'rusts' the arteries and veins, and start damaging the walls of body cells and organs.

According to the famous book by Keiichi Morishita: "Hidden Truth of Cancer" (Keiichi Morishita M.D., 1976), the body starts depositing acidic ash into the cells as the blood becomes acidic, to clean the blood and try and make it more alkaline. However, this makes the cells toxic and acidic and over time, a good number of these cells even die. There are, of course, some that do survive and adapt to the new environment. Put differently, instead of dying like the rest of the cells, they live on by becoming 'abnormal cells'. These kinds of cells are also known as 'malignant cells'. They don't correspond with the DNA memory code or the brain functions; they grow without order and the victim is diagnosed with cancer.

2: Mitochondrial dysfunction

Some experts in modern science also assert that cancer can begin in the mitochondria (or the power stations in the cells). A cancer cell is different from a normal, healthy cell.

Healthy cells usually produce energy in the mitochondria by a process (which actually entails over 20 steps) where the carbohydrate is burned to produce energy among other products. For hundreds of millennia, the mitochondrial process chemical reactions have become adapted to the use of potassium to make the mitochondria function more efficiently.

However, the average human body typically has more sodium than potassium, which means that if it were left to natural osmosis, the sodium would leak into the cells slowly and potassium would be leaked out. The sodium would therefore replace the potassium in the mitochondrial processes. This automatically means that the process will start using more sodium than potassium- which would definitely work, but with reduced efficiency. Generally, less oxygen would be burned and the energy produced as a result would be limited. In this case, you'd have more sodium salts waste- whose acidity is more than that of the potassium salts. The power stations' environment now has an acidity level that reduces the efficiency of the whole energy production process. Try looking at the power stations as tiny batteries which are running down, leaving very little energy to power the gene (p53 gene) that is responsible with the regulation of cell division. The battery however still has power (given the current conditions) to power other genes, which is something that sends the cell division out of control. When that happens to you, a downward spiral begins and you begin your journey to ill health, which may include cancer.

The reason healthy people don't experience this process is the simple fact that there are 'pumps' on the cellular membrane that push potassium into the cell while keeping sodium outside. This means that your diet should be made up of good amounts of potassium and magnesium; higher than sodium (which an alkaline diet provides) to give you healthy and predominantly alkaline cells.

Unfortunately, most people eating the western diet end up taking in a lot of sodium and very little potassium and magnesium due to the nature of the diet or the foods it entails. The alkaline is the life-saver we all need because it provides enough potassium and magnesium to keep you away from cancer by ensuring your mitochondria are functioning right.

Acidity and heart disease

Undeniably, heart disease is one of the leading causes of death in America. This therefore makes it quite important to understand the relationship between heart disease and blood acidity.

When the healthy alkaline balance of the body is disturbed, it can affect the arteries in a number of ways. To begin with, when blood turns acidic, the electrical charges on the outside of your red blood cells become altered, making them stick together like magnets. When your blood cells stick together this way, they have a higher chance of creating clots in your blood vessels, which can lead to strokes.

Excessive acidity can also harden your arteries- this condition is known as atherosclerosis. Most people think that cholesterol is the only problem when it comes to the formation of the deadly plaque inside blood vessels; hyperacidity and shifts in mineral concentrations in the tissues can also lead to this problem. You already know that when your body begins becoming acidic, minerals like calcium are drawn out of your bones, and the magnesium is drawn from the cartilage into the connective tissues, arteries and interstitial spaces to sort of buffer or neutralize the acid.

When these minerals react with normal levels of cholesterol in the blood, some calcified deposits are formed, and atherosclerosis develops as a result. These deposits may block the arteries and lead to a host of diseases and conditions, including heart disease, stroke and atherosclerosis.

Other experts argue that acid wastes cause heart disease when your body tries to entomb them safely in calcium deposits. When you consume acidic food for extended periods of time, acid particles linger in the blood, triggering the onset of cardiovascular disease by making 'bumps and scratches' within arteries. The cholesterol and calcium in the blood then 'bandage' these injuries. As you'd expect, the higher the levels of cholesterol in the blood, the thicker the 'bandage' and thus, the narrower the arteries become. This therefore explains why cholesterol blocks arteries and makes them hard (since cholesterol cannot stick firmly to perfectly smooth vessels). Cholesterol sticks to artery walls that have been pitted and scratched –in this case, by acid particles.

Now, when you have narrowed arteries, you are at risk of developing different conditions. As earlier mentioned, blood clots can develop (they can also be formed when fatty plaques detach from your artery walls) and travel to the brain vessels through the bloodstream and increase the risk of getting strokes. They can also raise your blood pressure and increase your risk of getting a heart attack and strokes as well.

This therefore means that you should focus on water and food that is rich in alkaline minerals like magnesium and potassium to neutralize acids in your blood and restore your body to optimum balance. When the acids are well neutralized, the whole process will prevent any more scarring of your blood vessels, removing the need for cholesterol to create a protective coating.

If you already have cholesterol deposits formed on your blood vessels, the process of alkalizing the body will assist to break them down and disperse them throughout your bloodstream and reduce the load placed on your cardiovascular system.

And that's not all; you need to note that the bad cholesterol (that causes blockages) in the blood is usually caused by foods that contain a high glycemic index (they have a high impact on your blood sugar levels, causing peaks within short periods of time) such as processed foods, simple-carbohydrate foods (like pasta and white rice) and sugary fast foods/treats, which are highly discouraged in the alkaline diet. Bad cholesterol can also be caused by saturated fats, found in red meats, trans-fats and foods prepared with shortening. These are also discouraged in alkaline dieting.

This study published in Jama Internal Medicine showed that such foods (especially the ones with a high Glycemic index) increase the levels of the bad cholesterol in the body and contribute to the risk of stroke and heart attack. (McMillan-Price J, 2006)

This is supported another study by Levitan (Levitan EB, 2008)

Bonus: Mental and emotional balance

Emotional balance is usually determined by the brain function. If your brain function is good, then your emotions are more likely to be balanced (or easier to balance).

The brain functions best when the body is fed with a sustainable fuel source, enough antioxidants, minerals and vitamins as these nourish it and protect it from oxidative stress- this is the damage (characterized by aging and neurodegenerative diseases) caused when your body is unable to neutralize elements known as free radicals produced in the body due to a lack of enough antioxidants. The alkaline diet is perfect for the brain because it provides all these nutritional components that nourish and protect the brain.

Secondly, we've talked at length about sugar and insulin. It turns out that these are some of the most important factors that control emotional balance. Insulin is a master growth regulator, which orchestrates the activity of many other hormones such as aldosterone, which regulates blood pressure, testosterone and estrogen which manage reproduction and stress hormones like adrenaline and cortisol. In this case, each time your insulin spikes or becomes imbalanced, most of these hormones become imbalanced as a result, affecting your mood, appetite, blood pressure, energy and concentration- just to mention the least.

Don't forget that what causes an imbalance in insulin levels is refined and processed carbohydrates, which most of us are used to consuming all the time, thus causing multiple insulin spikes each day, and a hormonal roller coaster all day long (which continues even when you sleep); as a result, you pay the emotional price. You feel fatigued, experience mood swings, bouts of irritability, insomnia, anxiety, lack of focus, and at times, depression. Following a diet that balances your sugar levels and insulin levels is obviously the way to go.

Third, there was a research paper (Adam E. Ziemann, 2009) published in Cell that suggested a link between pH and panic and anxiety. According to the paper, the amygdala is a chemosensor that detects acidosis, leading to 'fear' behavior. The researchers were mostly interested in a protein known as ASIC1a (Acid Sensing Ion Channel 1a) which is essentially acid sensitive. When the fluid around the nerve cells expressing this protein become acidic, they are activated.

One of the most common causes of acidosis (according to the study) is an increase in Carbon dioxide in the body- which the body is unable to take care of in good time. The levels of this gas rise and it is converted to carbonic acid in the blood.

Research proves that the amygdala, a brain part that is involved in anxiety, fear and panic (among many other functions), contains a lot of ASIC1a. This means that when carbonic acid increases and is not addressed, or even any other form of acid (or acidosis) in the blood, you may have anxiety and panic. This is especially true and worse if you are vulnerable to panic attacks. Having a diet that is always working to maintain a pH balance in your body at all times is one of the best solutions. The alkaline diet will therefore prevent acidity in your brain, and consequently, any possible emotional imbalance.

Summary (The Importance of Maintaining the Right pH Balance In The Body)

Having the right pH balance in the body helps in:

- Reducing the risk of developing degenerative diseases and the risk of diseases like renal failure sepsis, lung disease and obstructive lung disease.

- Reducing insulin resistance, thus reducing the likelihood of developing diabetes or gaining excess weight.

- It leads to a better control of cortisol, which improves the memory function, energy and immunity and prevents the following:

  - ✓ Reversing impaired cognitive function

  - ✓ Fighting reduced bone density

  - ✓ Fighting suppressed thyroid performance

  - ✓ Dealing with hyperglycemia and other forms of blood sugar imbalances

  - ✓ Reversing increased blood pressure

  - ✓ Dealing with reduced muscle tissue

  - ✓ Dealing with reduced inflammatory responses in the body and lowered immunity

- Reducing the risk of developing cancer and helps in its management through better mitochondrial function and countering the damaging effects of acidic ash.

- Reduce heart disease by reducing the hardening of arteries and blood clotting in blood vessels

- Improving mental and emotional balance by improving the brain function.

Breather

With what we've discussed so far in mind, you may be tempted to think that the aim of the alkaline diet is to increase the body's alkalinity so that it remains in an alkaline state. Unfortunately, that's not the case. Just to be clear, the aim of this diet is to balance your body's pH by reducing its acidity.

The human blood is an important medium and some kind of a vehicle that carries ions to different body parts. The total stability and optimal functioning of your body systems is therefore very important. In this light, your body is designed to maintain a really delicate pH balance in its tissues, fluids and systems. Given that most biochemical reactions critical in life occur in an aqueous environment, it means that it is your interstitial fluids and blood plasma surrounding the cells that are most sensitive to an imbalance between alkalinity and acidity- as they have a strict, varied pH range (which, in some organs even goes below 7).

It would be wrong to assume the body doesn't need some level of acidity therefore (by making it alkaline) because there are many processes/organs that depend on some level of acidity, including the following:

Stomach

There are digestive enzymes in the body that digest foodstuffs in the stomach; these enzymes have to be within a certain pH range to function optimally. Given that the stomach pH and that of the intestines determine the quality and rate of digestion, this is critical (otherwise you wouldn't benefit from the foods you eat). Therefore, your saliva (for instance) has to have a pH that is just below neutral for the digestive enzymes it contains to function optimally, control viral and bacterial growth and yield desirable health benefits.

In the stomach, there is the hydrochloric acid, which breaks down proteins (through a process known as proteolysis) and by activating an enzyme known as pepsin, it also facilitates chemical signaling for food to pass from the stomach to the ileum and also prevents the growth of bacteria that usually comes with food into the body, averting possible infection. If your body is too alkaline, all these functions and more would be affected and your body would experience a slow but massive systemic damage.

Your red blood cells are tasked with carrying oxygen to all the body cells to be used in respiration. When the pH in your blood is within the right acid-base balance, it becomes possible for the red blood cells to hold enough oxygen. If your body is too alkaline (usually way above 7.19- for the red blood cells), the red blood cells will not perform their role well. The alkaline diet principles appreciate the fact that the body pH is in a very tight range that's within a few tenths, and also that different illnesses can occur if the urine, saliva, blood etc. go far out of range.

As the last example, let's talk about bile acids. The liver has to have a certain level of acidity for bile acids to be secreted. Bile acids, contained in the chemical known as bile, modulate metabolism of glucose and lipids. They also control energy homeostasis. Just imagine what would happen if the body suddenly became alkaline!

There are many other areas in the body that require a slight level of acidity to function properly, even though the whole body environment is largely alkaline. It is therefore important to not offset the natural and required level of acidity in the body. The alkaline diet therefore works to maintain the right 'natural' balance between acidity and alkalinity in the body.

With that in mind, let's now discuss foods you can eat to achieve the alkalinity your body needs to perform optimally.

The Alkaline Diet Foods
(What To Eat And Avoid)

I know this is the part you had been waiting for. Without further ado, let's begin with the foods you should eat:

Eat These Alkalizing Foods

Alkalizing Vegetables And Grains:

Wild greens	Radishes	Mustard greens
Wheat grass	Pumpkin	Mushrooms
Watercress	Peppers	Lettuce
Tomatoes	Peas	Kohlrabi
Sweet potatoes	Garlic	Kale
Sprouts	Eggplant	Greens
Spirulina	Edible flowers	Green peas
Spinach	Parsnips	Green beans
Sea veggies	Onions	Quinoa
Rutabaga	Nightshade veggies	Amaranth

Millet	Cabbage	Daikon
Fermented veggies	Broccoli	Hemp seed oil
Dulce	Beets	Sunflower seeds
Dandelions	Alfalfa	Flax seeds
Cucumber	Wakame	Pumpkin seeds
Collard greens	Umeboshi	Chia seeds
Chlorella	Reish	Kamut
Chard greens	Nori	Spelt
Celery	Maitake	Rye
Cauliflower	Kombu	
Carrot	Dandelion root	

Alkalizing Fruits:

Watermelon	Rhubarb	Peach
Umeboshi	Raspberries	Orange
Tomato	Raisins	Nectarine
Tangerine	Plums	Muskmelons
Strawberries	Pineapple	Melon
Coconut	Pear	Lime

Lemon	Dried figs	Banana
Honeydew	Dates	Avocado
Grapefruit	Cherries	Apricot
Fresh currants	Cantaloupe	Apple
Dried grapes	Blueberries	

Alkalizing Protein And Nuts:

Whey protein powder	Millet	Hazelnuts
Tofu (fermented)	Eggs (especially egg whites)	Brazil nuts
Tempeh (fermented)	Chestnuts	Chestnuts
	Almonds	

Alkalizing Spices, Seasonings And Sweeteners:

Tamari	Miso	Chili pepper
Sea salt	Herbs (all)	Turmeric
Mustard	Ginger	Coriander
Agave	Curry	Paprika
Date sugar	Cinnamon	

Others

Spring water

Honey (use in little amounts)

Probiotic cultures

Alkaline veggie juices

Blackstrap

Alkaline antioxidant water

Apple cider vinegar
(use in little amounts)

Avoid These Acid- Forming Foods

Acidifying Vegetables, Grains And Grain Products

Lentils	Wheat	White beans
Cranberries	Spaghetti spelt	Soy milk
Corn	Rice cakes	Soy beans
Canned or glazed fruits	Macaroni noodles	Rice milk
	Crackers	Red beans
Wheat germ	Cornstarch	Pinto beans
Wheat flour	Bran	Lentils
Wheat bread	Barley	Kidney beans

Acidifying Dairy

Processed ice cream

Milk

Pecans

Ice milk

Peanuts

Butter cheese

Peanut butter

Acidifying Animal Protein

Venison	Sardines	Fish
Veal	Salmon	Corned beef
Turkey	Rabbit	Cod
Tuna	Pork	Clams
Shrimp	Pike	Carp
Shellfish	Oyster	Beef
Seafood	Organ meats	Bacon
Scallops	Mussels	
Sausage	Lamb lobster	

Acidifying Fats & Oils

Safflower oil

Corn oil

Lard

Canola oil

Acidifying Sweeteners

Sugar

Corn syrup

Maple syrup

Carob

Acidifying Alcohol

Wine

Hard liquor

Spirits

Beer

Other Foods

Soft drinks

Coffee

Mustard

Catsup

Looking at the list above, you might wonder why citrus foods aren't classified as acidic. While they contain varying amounts of citric acid, they usually have an alkalizing effect in the body system. In other words, they leave an alkaline ash when metabolized.

Again, you might also want to know that there are many versions of the alkaline diet food list. These lists usually have slight differences as regards to the classification of some foods. For instance, there are foods in the list above that have been classified as acidic that other charts will consider alkaline. However, there are only a few foods that are affected.

Lastly, you have to make sure you drink a lot of water. The water should be filtered and if possible, ensure it is spring water. Spring water is naturally alkaline. Therefore, make a daily target of taking 6-18 cups per day (but of course, you start slow and work your way up). If you are not the biggest fan of water, you can add some lemon to the water (1/4 lemon mixed with two cups of lukewarm is ideal). To make it even better and add variety, you can drink fresh juice (from the allowed fruits and vegetables list), make smoothies using the fruits and vegetables in the allowed list and even take herbal teas and drinks that I will discuss later in the book.

Let's now begin cooking!

Alkaline Breakfast Recipes

Scrambled Tofu

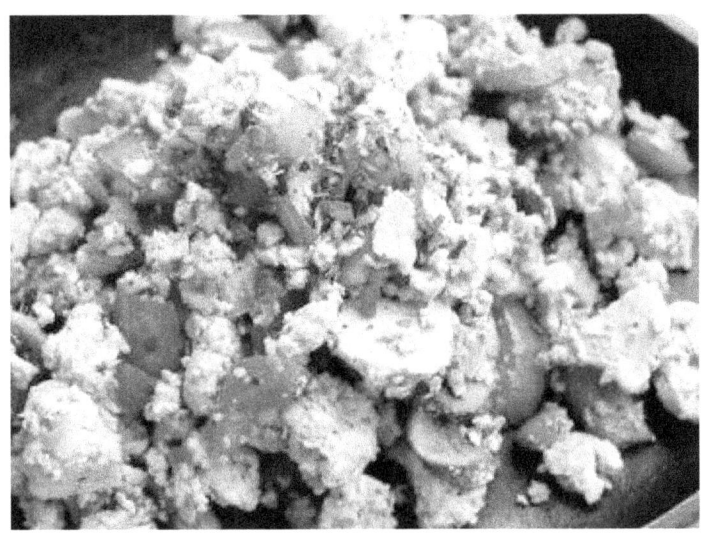

Yields 2 Servings

Ingredients

1 onion

3 tomatoes

1/2 teaspoon of cumin

1/2 teaspoon of turmeric

1 cup baby spinach

3 cloves

Some firm tofu

1/ teaspoon of paprika

1/2 cup of yeast

Salt for taste

Directions

Mince the garlic and dice the onion.

Add the onions to a pan and let it heat for 7 minutes. Add the garlic and cook for one more minute. Add the tomatoes and tofu and continue cooking for 10 minutes. Add the paprika, cumin and a bit of water, and stir well to cook.

Add the spinach at the very end.

Enjoy!

Millet Porridge

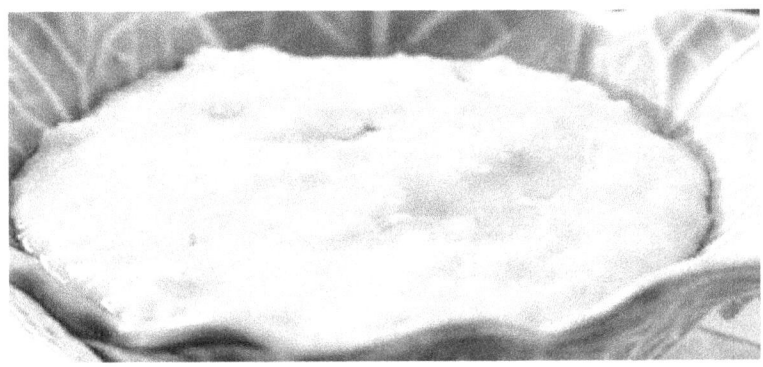

Yields 10 Servings

Ingredients

1 cup of millet

Pinch of salt

¼ cup agave syrup

10 cups of water

1 tablespoon of cinnamon

Directions

Add water to a large pot and bring to a boil. Then add the millet and salt.

Reduce the heat and cover with a lid then let it cook for 15 minutes before adding the cinnamon. Keep cooking the millet for 20 more minutes.

Add some agave syrup and keep stirring as you try to adjust the thickness.

Serve and enjoy when ready.

Super Seed Spelt Pancakes

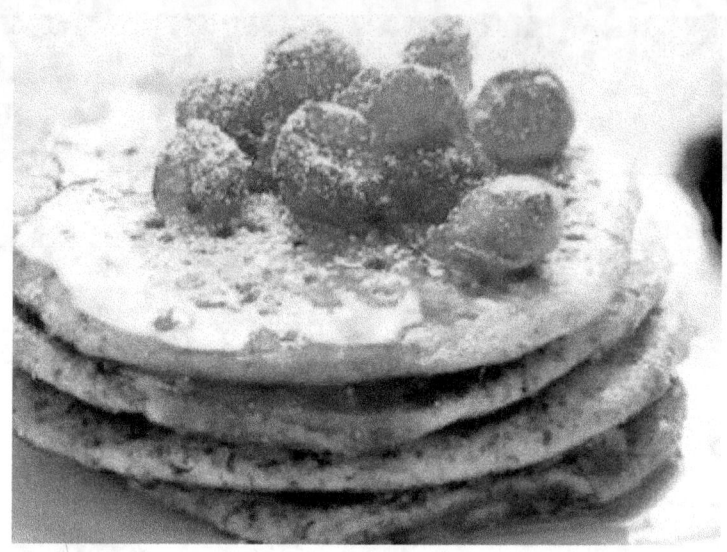

Yields 3 Servings

Ingredients

¼ cup pumpkin seeds

¼ cup flax seeds

1 cup quinoa or millet

1/2 teaspoon baking powder

1/4 teaspoon fine sea salt

2 tablespoon plant-based milk

¼ cup sesame seeds

1/2 tablespoon agave extract

½ cup chia seeds

1 1/2 teaspoons ground cinnamon

1 teaspoon baking soda

1 tablespoon coconut oil

Directions

Grind the chia seeds, pumpkin seeds, grouts, sesame seeds and flax seeds into a flour and store a quarter of the flour for later use as you won't need it here.

Add the 2 cups of the seed flour to a medium bowl and mix.

Add the rest of the ingredients apart from the coconut oil. You can add more milk if necessary to attain the right consistency.

Heat your pan with coconut oil and pour thin layers of the pancakes, flipping when you see bubbles appearing on top.

Keep doing this until you use up all the mixture.

Quinoa Porridge

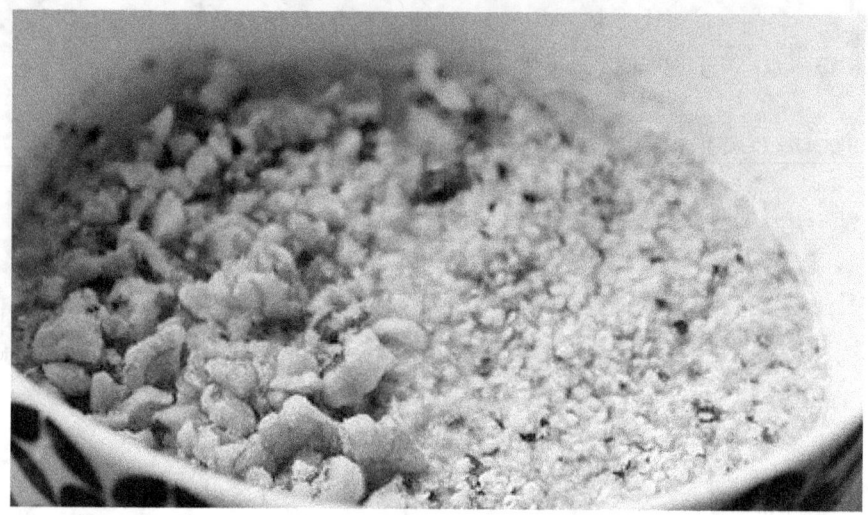

Serves 1

Ingredients

1/4 cup plant-based milk

1/2 cup quinoa flakes

1 tablespoon coconut oil

1 tablespoon chia seeds

¼ teaspoon ground cinnamon

Your favorite alkaline sweetener

Directions

Soak the chia seeds with three tablespoons of water overnight or for ten minutes.

Put the quinoa flakes into a pan containing 1 ¼ cups of water and then place on the stove top (or heat in the microwave).

Add the chia seeds, cinnamon, coconut oil and the sweetener and stir well until combined.

Top with crushed walnuts, hemp seeds or anything else you desire. Enjoy the dish with a green alkaline juice.

Soaked Almond and Seed Muesli

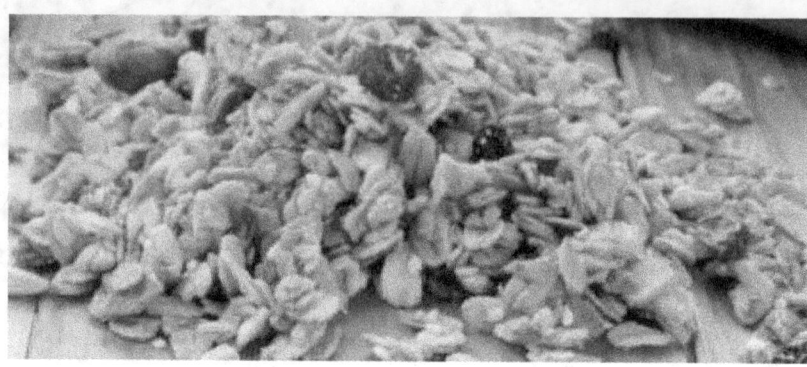

Yields 2 Servings

Ingredients

Cinnamon, to taste

1 tablespoon flaxseeds

1 tablespoon chia seeds

1 cup unsweetened almond milk

¼ cup raw pumpkin seeds

¼ cup raw almonds

Sweetener, to taste

Directions

Add all the ingredients to a bowl and season with cinnamon and a sweetener.

Soak overnight and enjoy in the morning.

Gourmet Breakfast

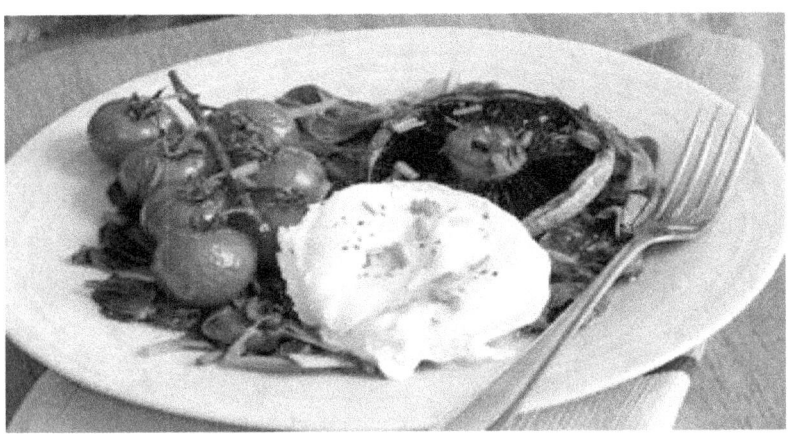

Yields 2 Servings

Ingredients

2 Portobello mushrooms

1 poached egg

1 cup sautéed spinach (salt and pepper added, to taste)

½ a dozen cherry tomatoes

Directions

Drizzle some olive oil over the mushrooms and tomatoes and season with a pinch of salt.

Grill or bake the tomatoes and mushrooms well until they're well cooked.

Add to a plate together with the egg and spinach.

Enjoy!

Cinnamon Quinoa

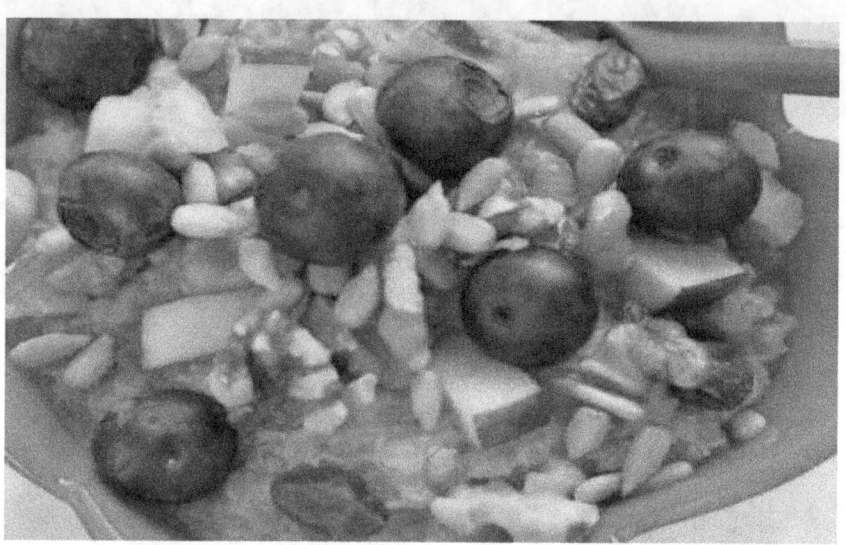

Yields 4 Servings

Ingredients

Agave, to taste

4 tablespoon raw sunflower seeds

3 cups unsweetened almond milk

1/4 teaspoon allspice

1/2 teaspoon vanilla

1/2 cup raw walnuts, chopped

1/2 cup raisins

1 teaspoon cinnamon

1 medium apple chopped into small slices (save some for garnish)

1 cup quinoa, rinsed

1 cup fresh organic blueberries, raspberries, fresh strawberries, chopped almonds, hemp seeds (optional)

Directions

Mix the almond milk, quinoa, cinnamon, raisins and allspice in a medium-sized sauce pan and bring to a boil.

Place a lid on the pan and reduce the heat to low.

After five minutes, add the apple pieces while stirring and let it simmer for between 5 and 7 seconds more.

Stir and then check whether the remaining liquid has been absorbed then remove from the heat but leave the lid on the pan, and then allow it to rest for five minutes to absorb the remaining milk. If you still see a lot of liquid when you peek, simmer for 3-5 more minutes, but make sure you keep a close eye over the pot as this mixture can easily burn if you leave it to boil dry.

Give it five minutes to rest, and then taste for sweetness.

Adjust with a few drops of agave. Just ensure you take care as the additional natural sugars can spike your blood sugar levels easily so go slow on them.

Serve and top with the sunflower seeds, walnuts, blueberries and the rest of the copped apple. You can also toss some strawberries and raspberries if using.

Blueberry Banana Smoothie

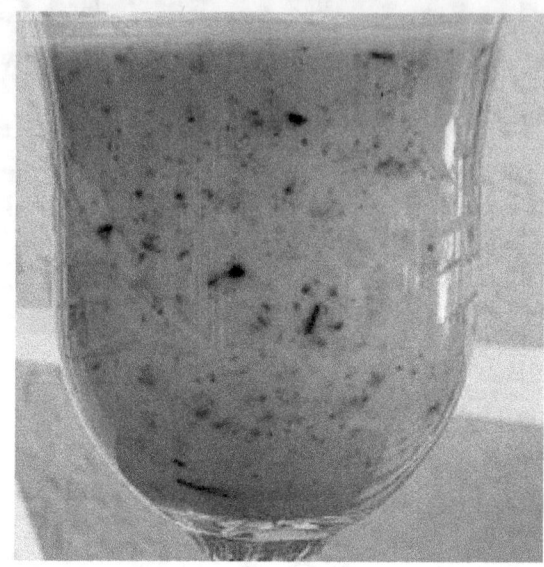

Yields 2 Servings

Ingredients

1 cup unsweetened almond milk

1 ripe banana large

1 scoop collagen peptides

1/2 cup blueberries preferably organic

2-3 tablespoons almond butter -preferably sprouted or soaked

1 splash vanilla extract (optional)

Directions

Add the ingredients to a wide-mouthed mason jar and mix well.

Add the mixture to a handheld blender and blend until smooth.

Serve immediately and store the leftovers in the refrigerator.

Note: If you are unable to source the sprouted/soaked almond butter where you live, you can look for a good brand of organic roasted almond butter instead.

Almond Flour Pancakes

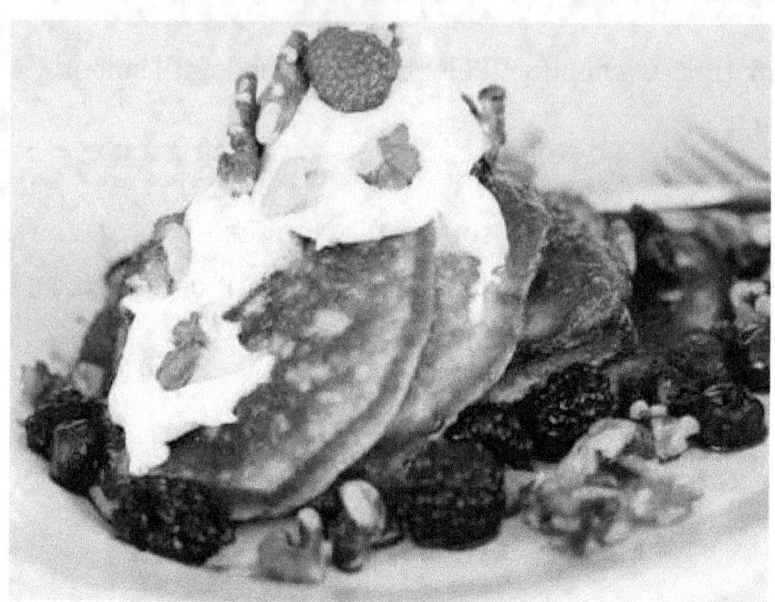

Yields 2 Servings

Ingredients

Sea salt, to taste

Coconut oil, for cooking

2 tablespoons agave syrup

2 eggs

1 cup almond flour

1/3 cup coconut milk

Directions

Add all the ingredients to a large mixing bowl apart from the coconut oil and mix using a wooden spoon until well integrated or until everything forms a batter.

Pour the coconut oil in a large skillet set over medium heat and heat.

Pour about ¼ cup of the batter onto a skillet and cook until bubbles appear on the surface of the pancake; this should take about three minutes.

When the bubbles appear, flip the pancakes using a rubber spatula and cook for 2-3 more minutes.

Add fresh berries, butter, whipped coconut cream, nuts, agave, cinnamon, a dab of agave, ghee and any other alkaline toppings.

Serve and enjoy!

Avocado Breakfast Bowl

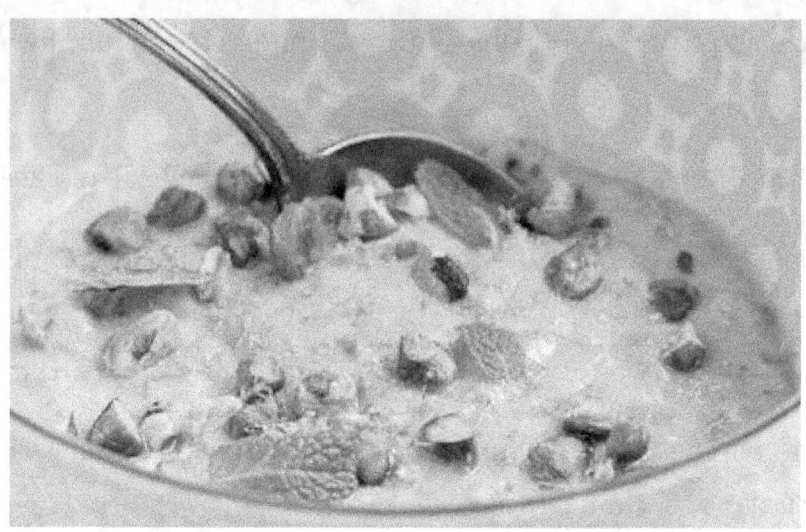

Yields 1 Serving

Ingredients

Pinch of sea salt

Juice of 1 lime

Chopped nuts, optional

Agave nectar, to taste

2 tablespoons melted coconut oil

18-24 fresh parsley/basil leaves

1/8 teaspoon lime zest, plus more for serving

1/2 cup cucumber, roughly chopped

1 avocado

Directions

Blend the avocado, sweetener and lime juice in a blender until smooth and creamy.

Add the chopped cucumber, sea salt, lime zest and coconut oil and then pulse a few more times until smooth and creamy.

Finally, add parsley or basil and blend until it just combines, and the herb is visible.

Serve the mixture in a serving bowl and top with chopped nuts such as Brazil nuts or walnuts and some lime zest.

Enjoy!

Homemade Ezekiel Bread

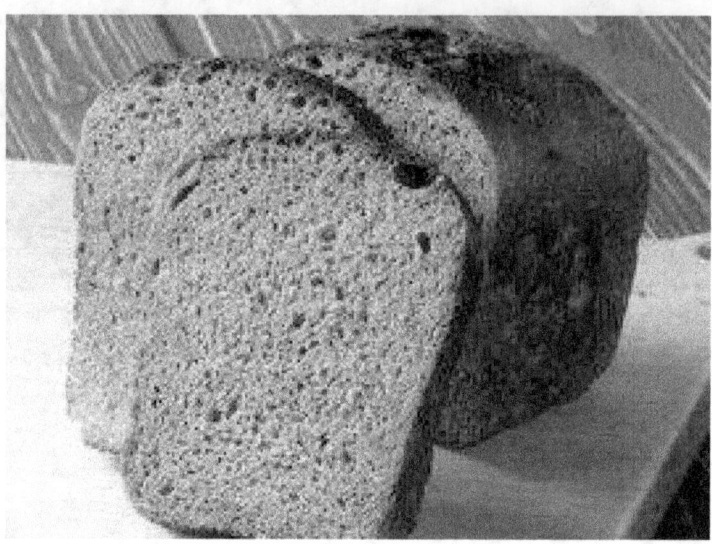

Yields 1 Bread

Ingredients

3 ½ cups sprouted wheat or millet, or a combination of your favorite sprouts

1 packet (1/4 ounces) dry-activated yeast

1 ½ teaspoon sea salt (Himalayan)

Directions

Place the sprouts in the oven or dehydrator and dehydrate for 12-18 hours. Dehydrate them or bake them (at very low temperature) at 115 degrees for the time stipulated above.

When they're fully dehydrated, place the sprouts in your food processor together with the salt and process until they form a ball.

Leave it in an airtight container for about 12 hours if you want a non-sourdough bread; otherwise, you can let it stay for 1 or 2 days for a nice, sour dough taste.

Knead the dough together with the dry-activated yeast for not less than 20 minutes.

Now form it into a ball and place it on a bowl. Cover with plastic and let it rise for 1-2 hours.

Preheat your oven to 350 degrees F.

Treat a bread pan with coconut or olive oil, add the dough and bake it for one hour.

Enjoy!

Portobello Mushroom Patties

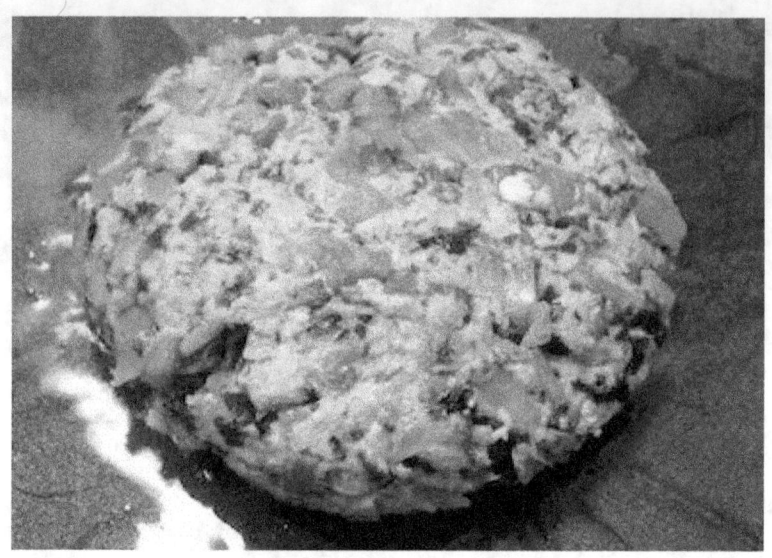

Yields 1 Serving

Ingredients

2 Portobello mushrooms

1/4 teaspoon oregano (dry/ fresh)

1/4 cup of cilantro

2 teaspoon onion powder (or red onion)

1/4 teaspoon sea salt, to taste

1/4 cup of flour (spelt, rye)

1/2 cup bell peppers (red /green)

1 Pinch of cayenne pepper

Directions

Add the mushrooms to some water for one minute to soak, and then process them together with the bell peppers and scallions in a food processor. If you don't have a food processor near you, dice up the peppers and mushrooms.

Combine the ingredients properly to form a patty.

Add the flour and seasonings; combine again to form patties and then add each one of them to a heated pan along with two tablespoons of oil, frying both sides until they're done; they should each take roughly three minutes to cook.

Apple Cinnamon Muffins

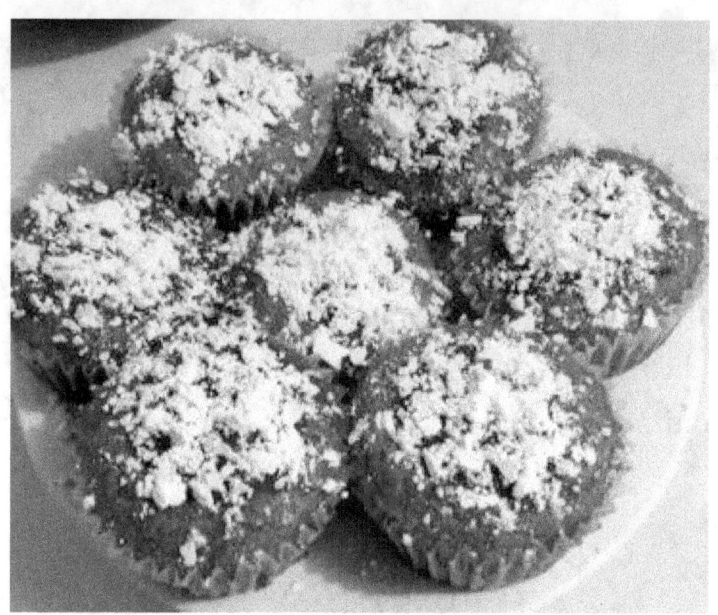

Yields 12 Muffins

Ingredients

<u>For the muffins</u>

1 3/4 cups spelt flour

1 tablespoon baking powder

1 teaspoon ground cinnamon

4 ounces coconut milk

2 tablespoons agave nectar

3/4 cup coconut sugar

1/2 teaspoon salt (pink Himalayan salt)

8 ounces applesauce

4 ounces coconut oil or other alkaline oil of your choice

For the topping

1 teaspoon cinnamon

2 tablespoons coconut sugar

Directions

Preheat your oven to 400 degrees F. In the meantime, line a muffin tray properly and set aside.

Add the baking powder, flour, cinnamon, sugar to a large bowl and stir well.

Get another bowl and add applesauce, agave nectar, coconut milk and oil; add the wet ingredients to the dry ones and stir well until well combined.

Add the mixture to the muffin cups (until they're 2/3 full) and then add some sugar and a sprinkle of cinnamon.

Bake for 18 to 20 minutes and allow it to cook for 20 minutes in the pan.

Transfer the muffins to a cooling rack to complete the cooling.

Enjoy!

Spelt Alkaline Waffles

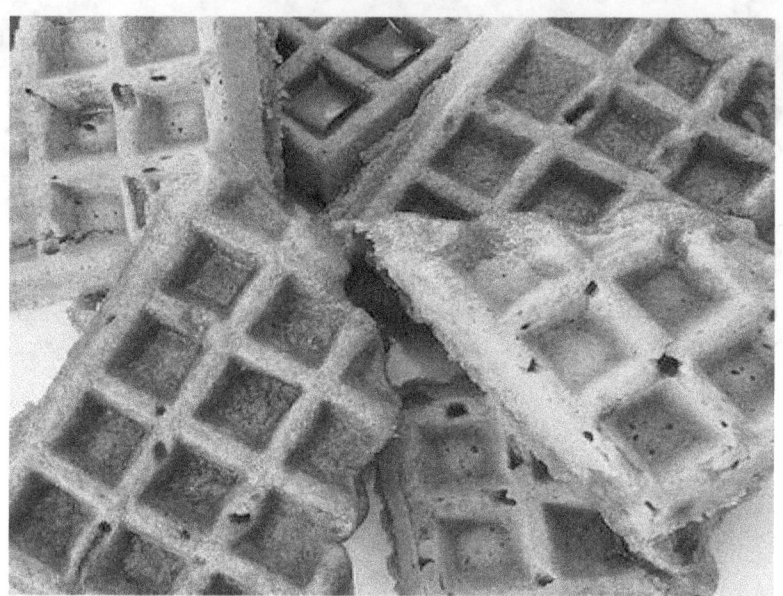

Yields 2 Servings

Ingredients

2 ½ cups spelt flour

½ teaspoon sea salt

1 cup spring water

3 tablespoons date sugar

1 ½ cups of hemp milk

3 tablespoons hemp seed oil

Directions

Add the sugar, flour and salt to a large mixing bowl and mix together.

Add the oil, water and milk and stir together until well integrated. You want to have a thick batter.

Preheat your waffle maker on any setting you prefer (you can use 3 if unsure) and then brush once with oil.

When the machine is ready for use, add ½ cup batter to the center and start cooking. The waffles should be ready when the green light shows.

Repeat the process with the rest of the batter and serve warm with a drizzle of agave cactus syrup.

Chia Porridge with Berries, Nuts and Seeds

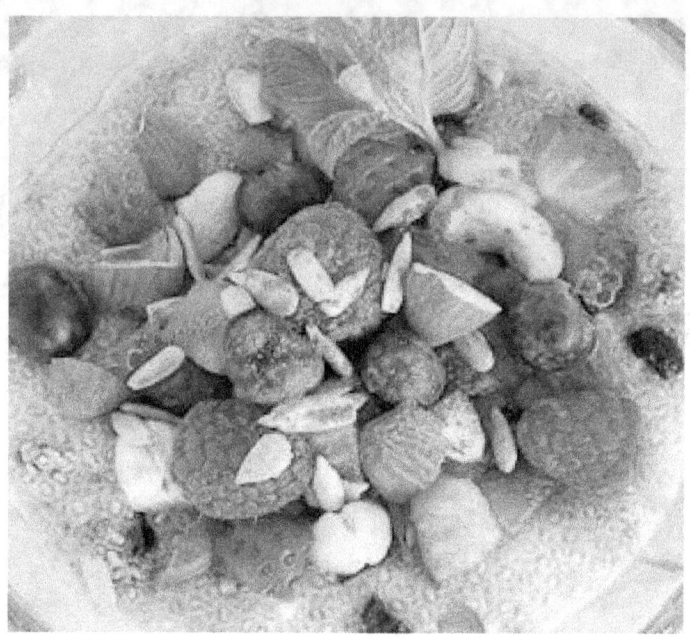

Yields 1 Serving

Ingredients

3 tablespoons chia seeds

2 tablespoons dried organic berries of choice

1/4 teaspoon all spice

1/2 teaspoon vanilla

Additional diced strawberries, raspberries & blueberries for toppings

1 cup organic almond milk

1/2-1 teaspoon cinnamon

1/8 teaspoon cardamom

3 drops liquid agave

Raw almonds, sunflower seeds and cashews for toppings (you can try using ones that have been soaked overnight for the best results)

Mint to garnish or use as topping

Directions

Add the almond milk and a sprinkle of chia seeds to a bowl and immediately begin stirring for one minute or so - to avoid any clumping.

Add the spices and berries as you stir, and then add the vanilla and three drops of agave sweetener; continue stirring a bit and leave it to sit for 30 to 40 minutes so that the mixture becomes thick.

Alternatively, you can cover it and put it in the fridge; let it stay there overnight before you serve.

To serve, add the nuts, berries, seeds and a sprig of mint.

Enjoy!

Aloha Smoothie

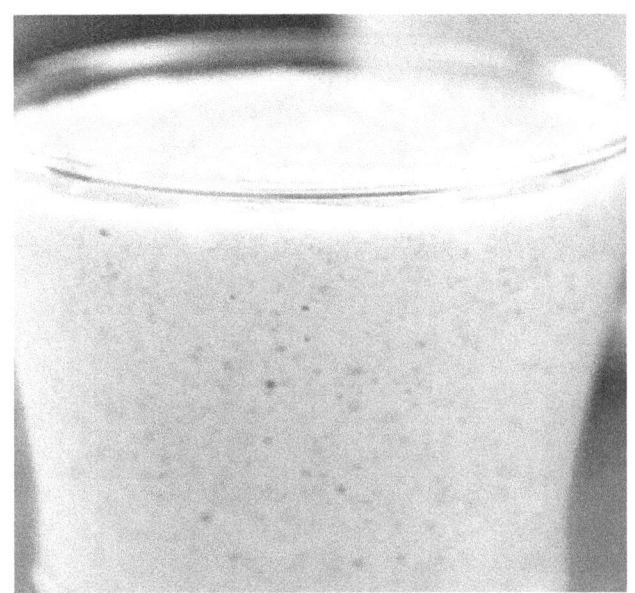

Yields 2 Servings

Ingredients

1 avocado

1/2 cucumber, chopped

Red grapefruit, peeled

Ice (if desired)

2 handfuls spinach

1-inch fresh ginger root

1/2 cup coconut water

Directions

Add all the ingredients to your blender and blend until smooth and creamy.

Enjoy!

Alkaline-Boosting Smoothie

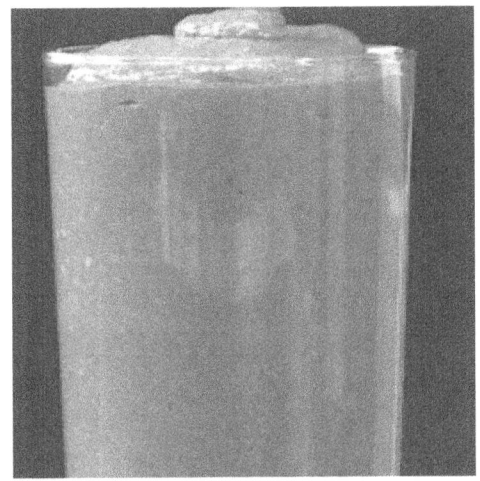

Yields 1 Serving

Ingredients

1/4 cup coconut milk

1 handful spinach

1 kiwi fruit

1/2 banana

1/4 cucumber

A handful ice cubes

Directions

Add the ingredients to a blender, and then blend until smooth and creamy.

Enjoy!

Alkaline Lime Smoothie

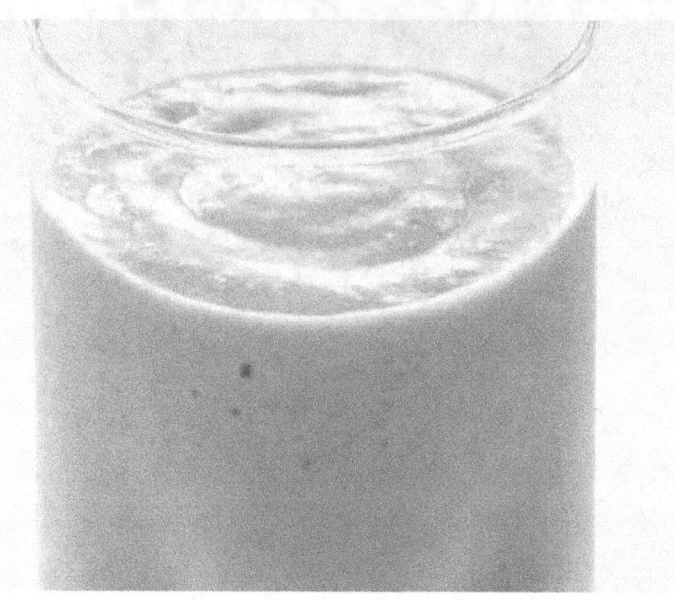

Yields 2 Servings

Ingredients

Pinch natural salt (optional, to bring out flavors)

Sweetener, to taste

2 tablespoons finely grated lime zest

2 limes, peeled and halved

2 cups firmly packed baby spinach

1 medium avocado, pitted and peeled

1 ½ cups ice cubes

¾ cup coconut water or water

½ medium cucumber, chopped

½ cup young Thai coconut meat- you can also use 1 tablespoon creamed coconut

Directions

Add all the ingredients to a blender and process for 30 to 60 seconds or until smooth and creamy.

Spinach & Strawberry Smoothie

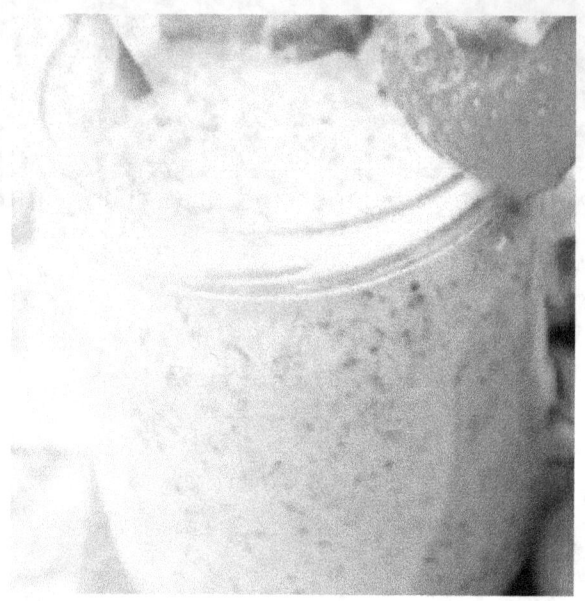

Yields 2 Servings

Ingredients

Juice from 2 oranges

225 grams strawberries

470 milliliters almond milk

240 grams natural yoghurt

45 grams spinach

Directions

Chop the de-stemmed strawberries and add them to a blender along with the other ingredients. Process until smooth and creamy.

Mint Kiwi Smoothie

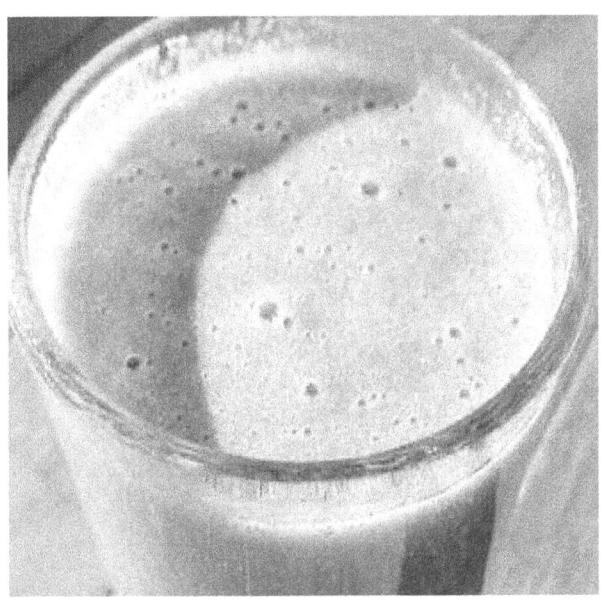

Yields 2 Servings

Ingredients

About 1 ½ cups fresh coconut milk

About ¾ cup cucumber, diced

2 medium kale leaves

2 medium frozen banana, chopped

2 full sprigs fresh mint

2 average sized kiwi, whole, but without ends

1/8 teaspoon sweetener

1 teaspoon hemp hearts

1 sprig top fresh basil

1 small avocado

1 cup ice, optional

Directions

Add all the ingredients to a blender and process until smooth and creamy

.

Alkaline Green Smoothie

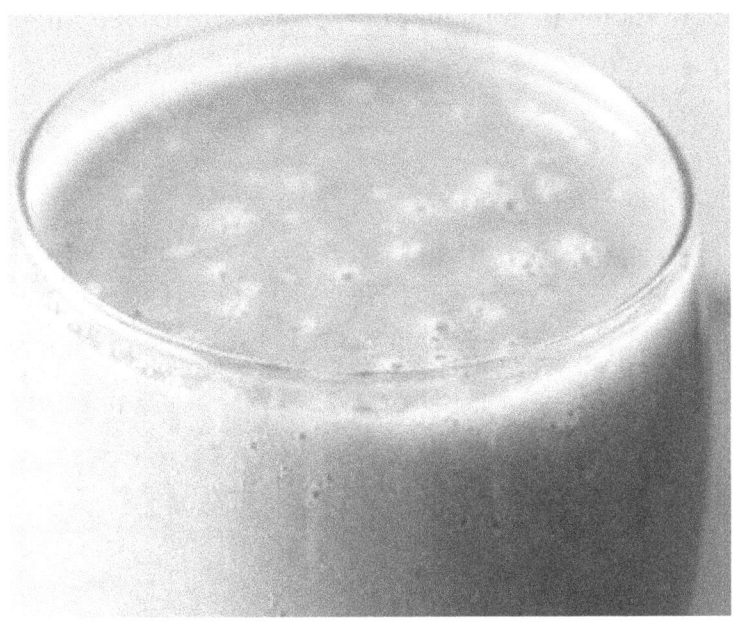

Yields 1 Serving

Ingredients

1/4 cup sliced frozen peaches

1/4 cup parsley

1/2 cup purified water

1/2 of one cucumber

Juice of 1/2 lemon

1 medium banana

1 cup packed organic spinach

8 ice cubes

Directions

Add all the ingredients to a blender and process until well integrated.

Ginger Green Smoothie

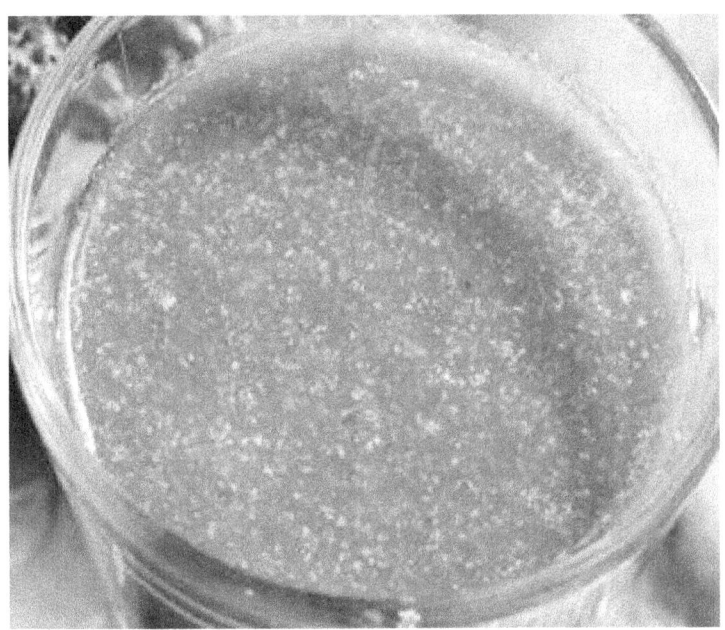

Yields 2 Servings

Ingredients

2 cups filtered water

1 frozen banana

1 tablespoon fresh ginger

4 cups spinach

2 cups frozen pineapple

½ lemons freshly squeezed

Directions

Add the greens and water to your blender and process until smooth.

Add the pineapple, ginger, banana and lemon juice. Process on high speed then serve immediately.

Alkaline Lunch Recipes

Broccoli Mushroom Rotini Casserole

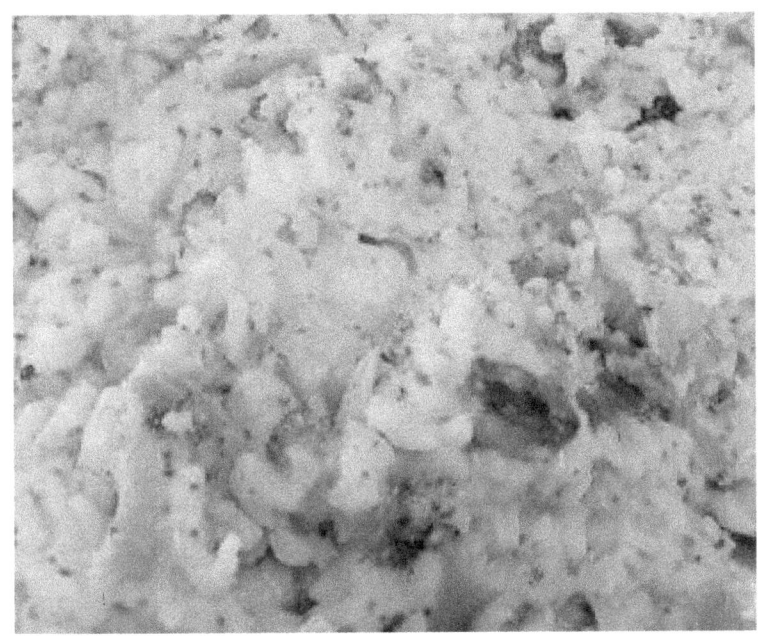

Yields 6 Servings

Ingredients

White pepper, to garnish

Paprika, to garnish

Herbamare or salt, to garnish

8 ounces sliced mushrooms

3 large garlic cloves

16 ounces whole wheat rotini

1/4 cup panko bread crumbs

1/2 teaspoon dried oregano

1/2 teaspoon dried basil

1 medium onion, peeled and quartered

1 cup of broccoli

Cheesy Sauce:

5 teaspoon brown rice miso paste

2 cups of almond milk

1/3 cup nutritional yeast

1 teaspoon smoked paprika

1/4 cup cashews

1 tablespoon alkaline cornstarch substitute (such as ground flaxseed)

1 large clove of garlic

Directions

Preheat your oven to 350 degrees F and bring a large pot of water to a boil; you can add some salt if you want.

Cook the spirals/rotini for 6 or so minutes or until just cooked (make sure you don't overcook it).

Add the garlic, onions, mushrooms and broccoli to a food processor and pulse until they break down into tiny pieces.

Now add the mixture to a sauté pan or a large wok and cook for 7 minutes or until they turn soft.

You can add some vegetable broth or water as necessary to cook.

Add the cheesy sauce ingredients to a blender and pulse.

Taste and adjust the seasonings as desired with more pepper and salt, or smoked paprika.

Drain the rotini and put it on the sauté pan; pour some sauce over it (you can also mix it in a large pot if you don't have enough room).

Toss well to coat.

Add the dish to a large casserole pan and top with smoked paprika and panko breadcrumbs.

Bake for about 20 - 25 minutes and then serve and enjoy.

Millet Tabbouleh

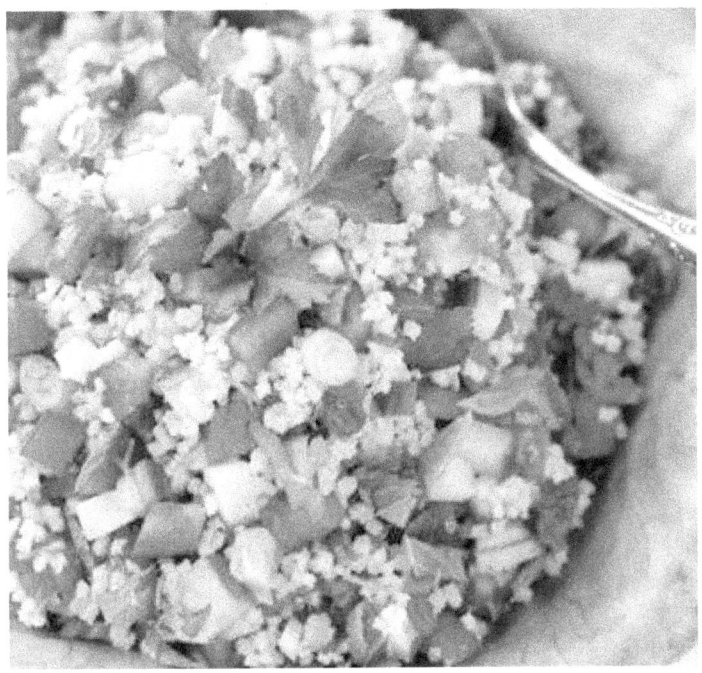

Yields 7 Cups

Ingredients

1 cup millet, rinsed

1 teaspoon Celtic sea salt

Juice of 1 lemon

1 1/2 cups of roma tomatoes, diced

3 green onions, sliced finely

3/4 cups of freshly chopped mint

2 cups filtered water

1/3 cup extra virgin olive oil

1/2 teaspoon Maldon sea salt flakes

1 large garlic clove, ground

1 1/2 cups of freshly chopped parsley

1 1/2 cups of diced English cucumber

Directions

Add water to a medium sized pan and bring it to a boil.

Add the millet and reduce the heat to low; cover and simmer for 18 – 20 minutes.

Now fluff using a fork and let it cool (without the lid for half an hour to one hour). It should have a firm texture (not crunchy or mushy).

Mix the lemon juice, crushed garlic and olive properly and let it stand.

In the meantime, chop the vegetables as per the descriptions above and add to a large bowl.

When the millet cools completely, add it as well and pour the dressing over the mixture, tossing the seasoning with sea salt to taste.

To serve, garnish with mint or parsley and enjoy!

You can serve either chilled or at room temperature. Also, the flavors will become a lot more pronounced if you allow it to rest for a little while.

Kale and Golden Beet Salad

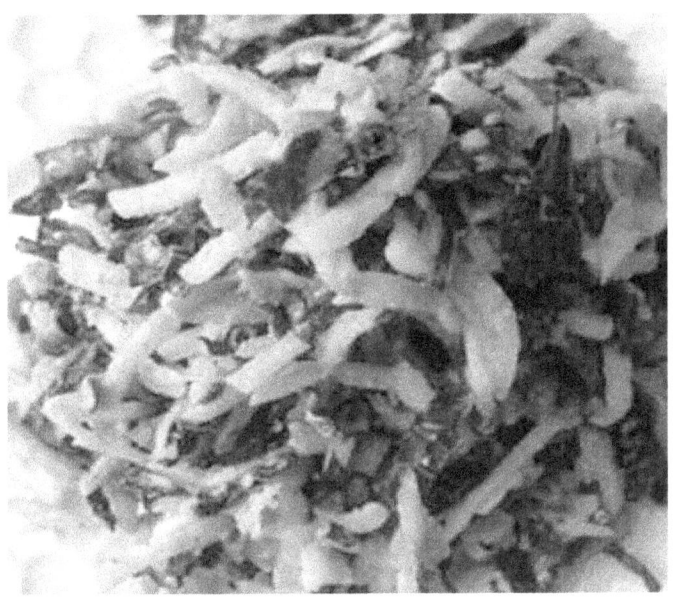

Yields 8 Servings

Ingredients

<u>Salad</u>

4 medium golden beets

4 green onions, bias cut

2 medium carrots

1 yellow bell pepper

1 bunch kale, without stems and cut into thin strips

<u>Dressing</u>

3 tablespoons tahini

3 minced garlic cloves

2 ounces coconut oil

2 ounces apple cider vinegar

1-inch piece of ginger, peeled and minced

1 teaspoon dried basil

1 tablespoon tamari

½ lemon, juiced

Ingredients

For the salad-

Add the green onions and kale to a large bowl.

Add the carrots, beets and bell pepper to a food processor and process. You can also do it by hand if you want.

Add the grated vegetables to the onions and kale mixture, and toss well to mix.

For the dressing-

Add the dressing ingredients to a small bowl and combine well. A hand-held emulsion blender is best used for here as it makes the mixture smoother and creamier.

Now pour the dressing over the salad ingredients and mix properly. Let it chill for not less than one hour before you serve (for the best flavor).

Watermelon Avocado & Raspberry Salad

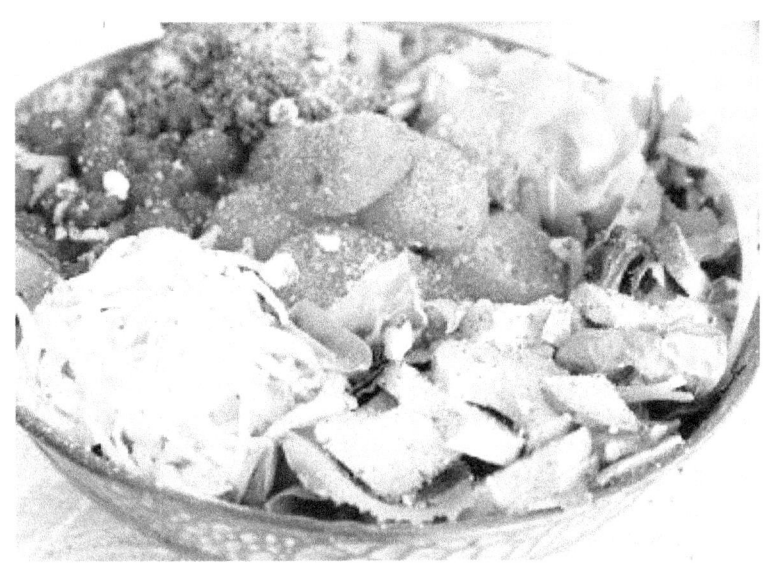

Yields 5 Servings

Ingredients

Salad

1/2 cup raspberries

1/2 cup toasted almonds

1 cup watermelon

1 cup baby broccoli

4 cups baby kale

1 cup cucumber sliced or spiral

1 sliced avocado

1 cup papaya

Dressing

1/4 cup goji berries

1/2 cup olive oil

1/2 cup master tonic (see recipe below)

Pinch sea salt

4 dates

Master tonic

Juice of 1 lemon

32 ounces organic apple cider vinegar

2 tablespoon horseradish, minced

2 knobs turmeric, chopped

1/4 cup onion, chopped

1/4 cup garlic, minced

1/4 cup fresh ginger, chopped

1 jalapeno pepper, chopped

Directions

For the salad

Combine the ingredients well apart from the almonds.

For the dressing

Combine the master tonic, olive oil and some salt until well integrated. Add the goji berries and dates to your blender and pulse until smooth.

Drizzle the dressing over the salad and complete the process with a sprinkle of the toasted almonds.

For the master tonic

Add the master tonic ingredients to some apple cider vinegar and blend the ingredients until they combine well.

Allow the tonic to set in a jar for 1-2 weeks, but shake it periodically.

Strain the ingredients and add the rest of the vinegar mixture to a jar and cover it.

You'll use this tonic in any salad dressing.

Brussels Sprout And Almond Salad

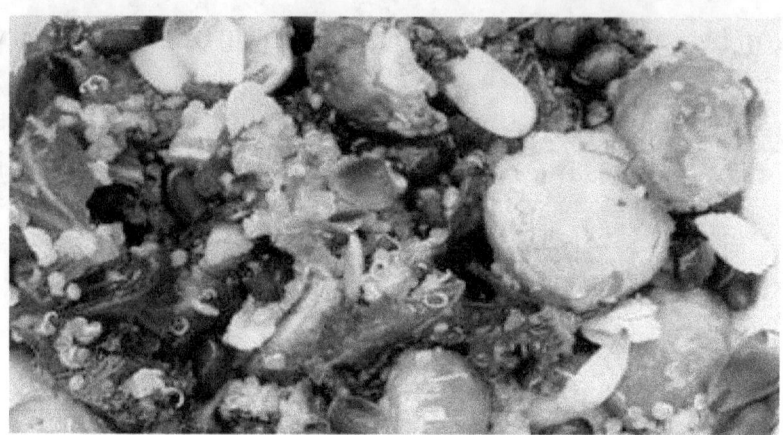

Yields 4 Servings

Ingredients

250g Brussels sprouts

100g kale

½ pomegranate

100g quinoa

3g fresh ginger

1 clove finely chopped garlic

30g flaked almonds

10g chopped fresh parsley

Zest of 1 orange

1 tablespoon olive oil

Pomegranate molasses

Directions

Preheat your oven to 175 degrees C. or 350 degrees F. and start preparing the sprouts.

Chop the base of the Brussels and then cut it in half.

Place them on a baking tray and add chopped garlic and a pinch of Himalayan salt over the top.

Bake them for 25 minutes.

Prepare the quinoa based on the packet instructions. Drain.

Chop the kale into chunks each measuring 3 inches and add them to salted boiling water for between 30 and 40 seconds. Strain.

Place the roasted Brussels sprouts in a bowl along with the blanched kale and quinoa.

Mix in the olive oil, orange zest, fresh ginger, fresh parsley and pomegranate molasses.

Add the flaked almonds to a pan and brown them for one minute over low heat; remove from the heat.

Add the pomegranate seeds- you can do this by holding the half in your hand such that the sliced side faces your palm; using a wooden spoon, bang the top so that the seeds fall out without their piths.

Serve the dish cold or hot and garnish with the flaked almonds and pomegranate seeds.

Spaghetti Squash Patties

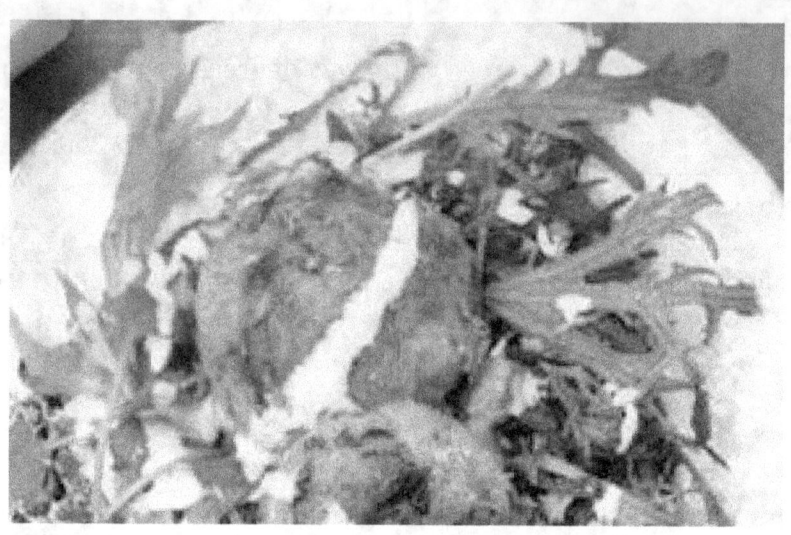

Yields 2 Servings

Ingredients

1 spaghetti squash

1 spring onion

3g fresh coriander

10g oat flour (optional)

1 teaspoon coriander

¼ teaspoon za'atar (spices)

4g grated ginger

1 teaspoon ground flax seed

30g finely chopped leeks

2 tablespoons sunflower oil

<u>Dressing</u>
3 tablespoons tahini

1 lemon juice

5 tablespoons water

Pinch of Himalayan salt

Directions

Preheat your oven to 350 degrees F. or 175 degrees C.

Cut the squash in half and lengthwise down the middle.

Scoop the seeds out and add 1 tablespoon of sunflower oil.

Place on the baking tray and bake for 40 minutes.

Allow it to cool and scoop out the insides using a fork. This will ensure the spaghetti strands are in place. Add them to a bowl.

Slice the leeks and spring onions thinly at an angle, and then add them to the squash, chopped coriander, grated ginger, ground coriander, ground flax seeds and za'atar.

Combine them together with the oat flour, if using and put it in the fridge to cool.

As it cools, add all the ingredients to a glass and whisk them together using a fork. If the mixture looks as though it's curdling, just continue mixing it until it forms a nice, smooth and creamy dressing.

If it is too thin, just continue adding tahini and a splash of water if it is too thick.

Add the remaining sunflower oil to a pan and heat.

When hot, create palm-sized patties with the squash mixture and place them on the pan carefully.

Sear them until they turn golden- this should take two minutes on each side.

Serve alongside the tahini dressing and green salad.

Quinoa Pasta with Tomato Artichoke Sauce

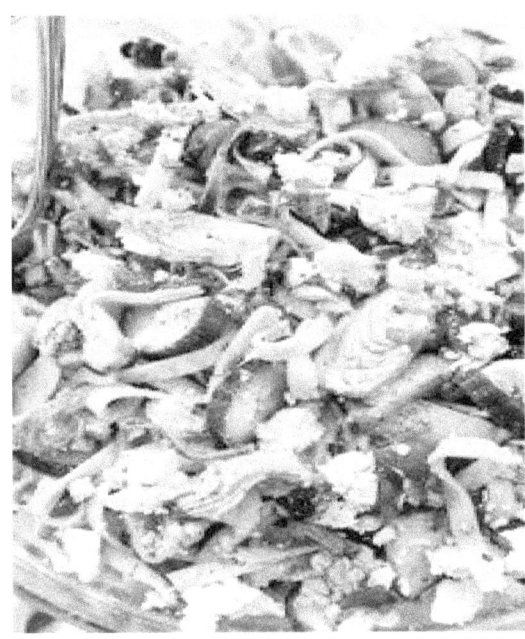

Yields 2 Servings

Ingredients

7 ounces quinoa or spelt pasta

5 ounces fresh tomatoes

1 clove garlic

1 teaspoon yeast-free vegetable stock

1/2 teaspoon organic sea salt

2 tablespoon cold-pressed extra virgin olive oil

8 ounces fresh or frozen artichoke hearts

1 medium-sized onion

1 ounce pine nuts

3 tablespoons fresh basil

1 pinch of cayenne pepper

Directions

Prepare the artichoke and cook it until soft and tender (you can also use frozen artichoke hearts here if you want).

Cook the pasta according to packet instructions. Cut the tomatoes into cubes and then chop the garlic, basil and onion into tiny pieces.

Add the olive oil to a pan and heat; stir-fry the onions, pine nuts and garlic for a few minutes and then add the tomatoes and cooked artichoke.

Stir-fry for two more minutes.

Add the yeast-free vegetable stock to ½ cup of water and then add to the pan. Simmer for two minutes on low heat, stirring occasionally.

Lastly, add the basil and season with salt and cayenne pepper.

To serve, drizzle the sauce over the cooked pasta. Serve immediately and enjoy!

Stir-Fry with Tofu & Coconut Milk

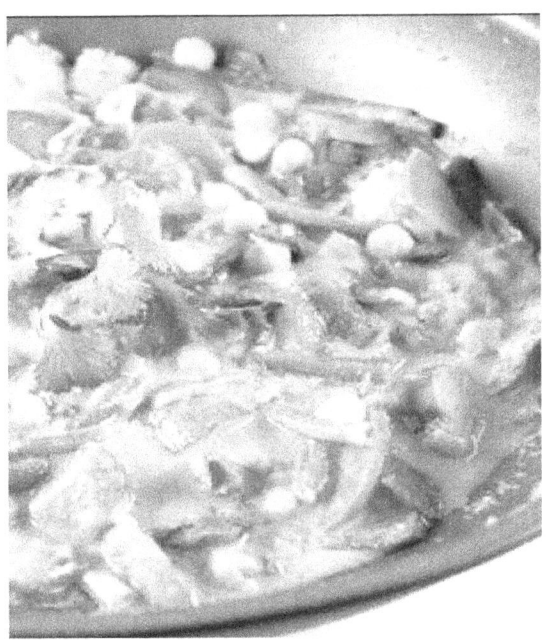

Yields 4 Servings

Ingredients

1 pound firm tofu

3 tomatoes

1 green pepper bell

1 to 1 ½ cups fresh coconut milk

Pinch of sea salt and pepper

¼ tablespoon ginger

3 medium-sized zucchinis

1 red pepper bell

½ pound green beans

2 tablespoons cold pressed extra virgin olive oil

½ tablespoons curry powder

Your favorite fresh herbs

Directions

Chop the zucchinis, pepper bells, beans and tomatoes, and dice the tofu into bite-sized pieces.

Add the oil to a wok or pan and fry the tofu for a couple of minutes.

Add the pepper bells, zucchini and beans and stir fry for a couple more minutes.

Then add the coconut milk and tomatoes, and stir properly for a few more minutes.

Season with ginger, curry powder, salt and your favorite herbs.

Serve with wild rice or soba noodles and enjoy!

Spanish Bean Salad

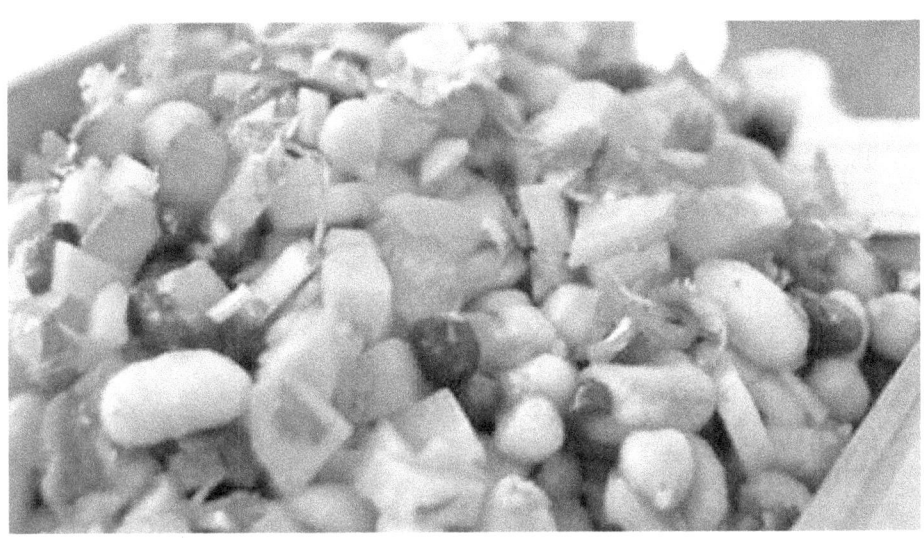

Yields 4 Servings

Ingredients

1/8 cup of chopped fresh cilantro

1/4 tablespoon of ground cumin

1/4 tablespoon of Celtic salt or sea salt

1/4 cup of olive oil

1/2 teaspoon of ground black pepper

1/2 tablespoon of hemp oil-optional

Cayenne pepper to season

1 carrot peeled & chopped

1 tablespoon of lemon juice

1 tablespoon of fresh lime juice

1 tablespoon of flax oil-optional

1 tablespoon of agave syrup

1 stalk celery, chopped

1 green onion, chopped-optional

½ teaspoon of chili powder

½ red bell pepper, chopped

½ can rinsed & drained pinto beans

½ can rinsed & drained chickpeas

½ can drained and rinsed cannellini beans

½ – 1 clove minced garlic

Directions

Mix the green onions, chopped veggies and beans in a large bowl and stir well to combine.

Add the rest of the ingredients to a large measuring cup and whisk them together to combine.

Now pour the dressing over the vegetables and combine them gently-ensure you don't mash the beans.

To serve, season with cayenne pepper and serve over fresh greens.

Sesame Mixed Vegetable Noodles

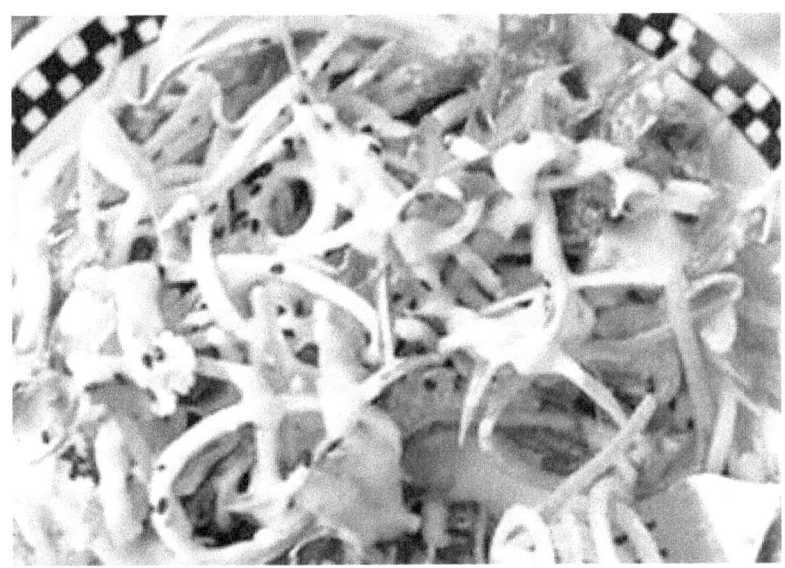

Serves 2

Ingredients

1/4 daikon radish, spiral noodle julienned or cut, about 1 to 2 cups

1/2 cup of carrots, julienned

1 cup of arugula

½ now peas, thinly slivered

1/4 bunch cilantro, chopped

1 small Patti /yellow zucchini pan, spiral noodle julienned or cut, about 1 cup

<u>The sauce</u>

1/2 cup of tahini, preferably raw

1/2 teaspoon of freshly grated ginger, optional

1/4 teaspoon toasted sesame oil, optional

1/8 cup of brags liquid Aminos

1/8 cup of juice of 1 lemon

1 tablespoon of filtered water

The garnish

Black or white sesame seeds for garnish

½ mango, thinly slivered

Directions

Mix the herbs and veggies in a large bowl and toss well.

Add the rest of the ingredients apart from the water to a measuring cup and combine until well integrated.

At this point, add some filtered water slowly until the mixture is smooth and creamy.

Toss the amount you need to serve —don't forget that the noodles and sauce keep well separately though.

Garnish with the mango, sesame seeds and the cilantro.

Enjoy!

Vegan Black Bean Chili

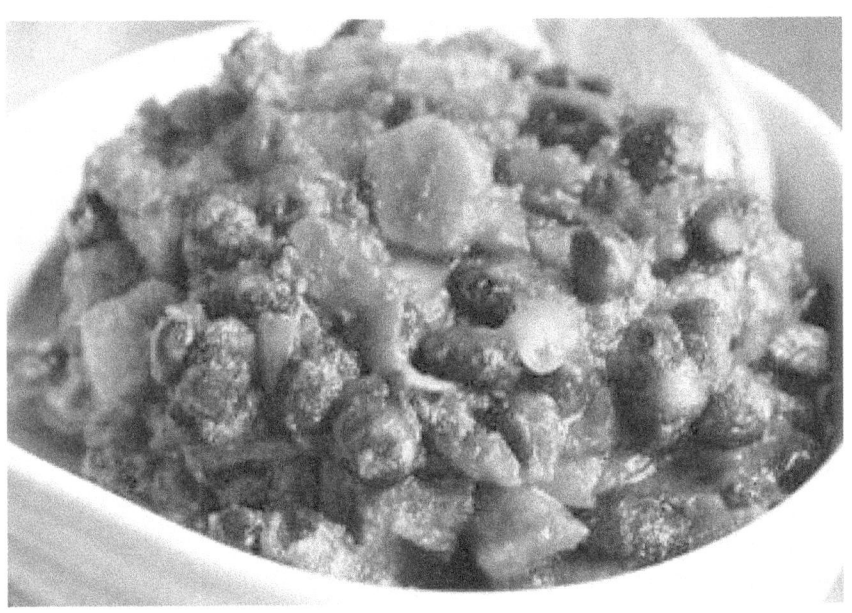

Yields 7 Servings

Ingredients

1 large onion, chopped

1 green bell pepper, seeded and chopped

1 can of organic crushed tomatoes

2 teaspoons (or more) chili powder

2 teaspoons smoked paprika

Salt to taste

Cilantro, chopped for garnish

2 large carrots, chopped

6 cups cooked black beans, drained

2 garlic cloves, peeled and sliced

2 teaspoons black pepper

2 tablespoons olive oil (you can also use vegetable broth- if oil-free)

Sweet potato chips (you can also use pear chips, apple chips or zucchini chips)

Directions

Add the oil or broth to a large soup pot (you can also use a Dutch oven) with a lid and heat until it shimmers.

Add the bell peppers, garlic, carrots and onion and cook for 3-5 minutes, making sure to stir occasionally until the mixture starts softening.

Add the rest of the ingredients and cook on low-medium heat for half an hour, uncovered. Ensure the chili only bubbles gently-it should not boil.

Now taste for spiciness and add more chili powder as desired, one teaspoon at a time (remember that chili powders usually vary in hotness).

It's easier to add spice gradually than end up with a too-spicy chili.

Cover the chili and let it "rest" on your stove's warm setting, or put it in the oven on warm for 30 minutes more.

Serve with sweet potato chips or zucchini chips, apple chips and pear chips, and garnish with chopped cilantro.

Vegan Alkaline Ribs

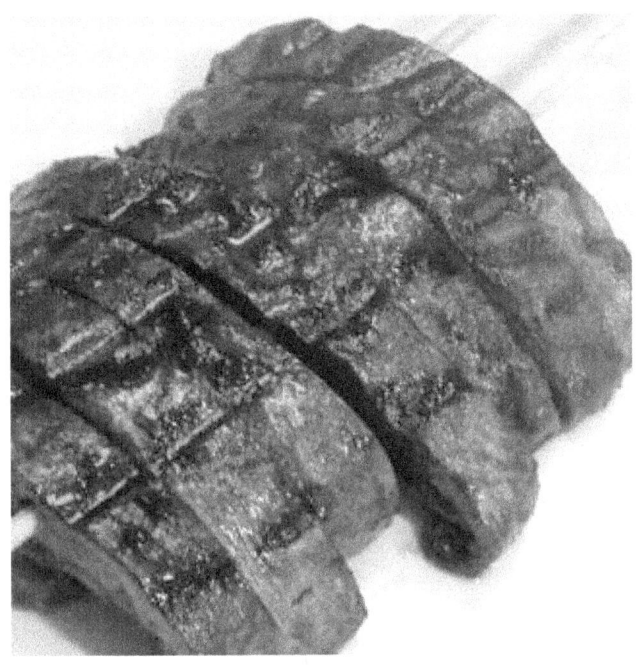

Yields 1 Serving (Per Mushroom)

Ingredients

2 Portobello mushrooms

1/4 cup spring water

1 teaspoon onion powder

Grape seed oil

1/2 cup Alkaline Barbecue Sauce

1 teaspoon sea salt

1/2 teaspoon cayenne

Basting brush

Skewers (optional)

Cast-iron griddle

Directions

Note: You can prepare this recipe on a grill, bake it at 350 degrees F for 10-15 minutes or cook using a skillet. Also, you can cook the mushrooms like 'riblets' if you don't have skewers.

So let's begin.

Scrape each mushroom's underside to remove the gills to get rid of any earthy taste.

Then slice the mushrooms roughly, ½ inch apart.

Get a large container and add the mushrooms along with water, seasonings and a huge portion of the barbecue sauce.

Cover with a lid and shake, and then store in the fridge for 6-8 hours- flip the container over after every 2 hours.

Push through three mushrooms around the middle of a skewer and then add 2-3 more slices to another skewer. In case any slices break, simply cook them as 'riblets'.

Brush the griddle with oil over medium heat and cook the ribs for 12 – 15 minutes, making sure to flip them every three minutes.

After every few flips, you can brush them with a bit more barbecue sauce if you want.

"Rice" with Fresh Peas and Cumin

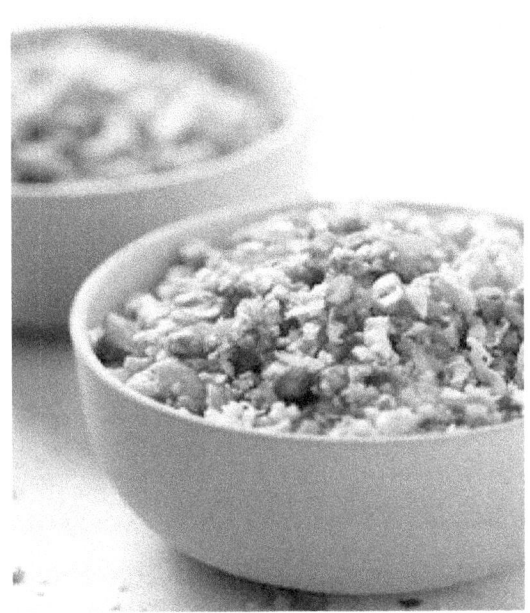

Yields 4 Servings

Ingredients

1 medium head cauliflower

4 scallions, thinly sliced

Zest from 1 lemon

2 teaspoons agave syrup

1/2 cup pine nuts

Pinch Himalayan salt and pepper

1 cup fresh peas

1/2 cup fresh lemon juice

2 teaspoons cumin

1 teaspoon grated fresh ginger

1 tablespoon chili flakes (optional)

Directions

Remove the cauliflower florets from the stems and then add to a food processor then process until the cauliflower breaks down into rice-sized pieces.

Add the scallions and peas while stirring.

Mix the lemon zest, lemon juice, ginger and agave syrup together and pour the mixture over the cauliflower mixture; stir to combine.

When the dish is ready, top with pine nuts and chili flakes and some salt/pepper to taste.

Enjoy!

Eggplant Rolls

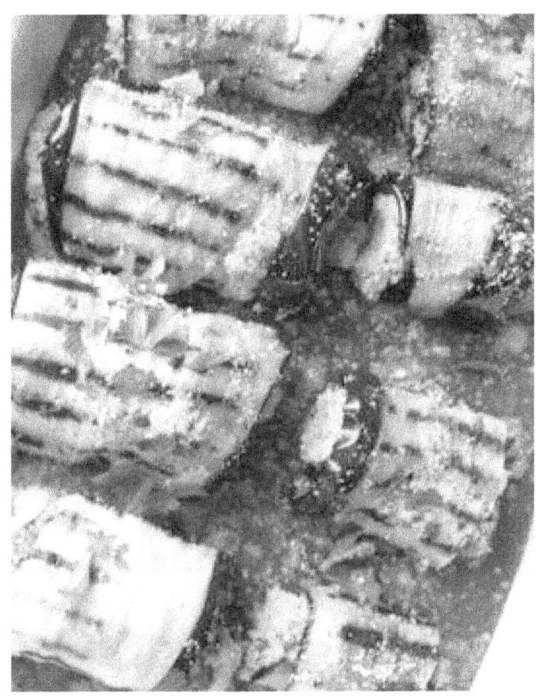

Yields 2 Servings

Ingredients

100 g eggplant

1g salt

1g oregano

10g olive oil

Directions

Start by cutting the eggplant lengthwise into long and thin slices, each measuring roughly ¼ inch.

Sprinkle oregano and salt on all the eggplant pieces lightly, front and back, and leave them for ten minutes.

Coat the pieces with a thin layer of olive oil and place them on a hot skillet set over medium-high heat.

Flip them over when the eggplant turns lightly brown, for about 2 minutes for each side.

Get the eggplant out of the skillet and roll it width-wise.

Enjoy!

Rice Paper Rolls

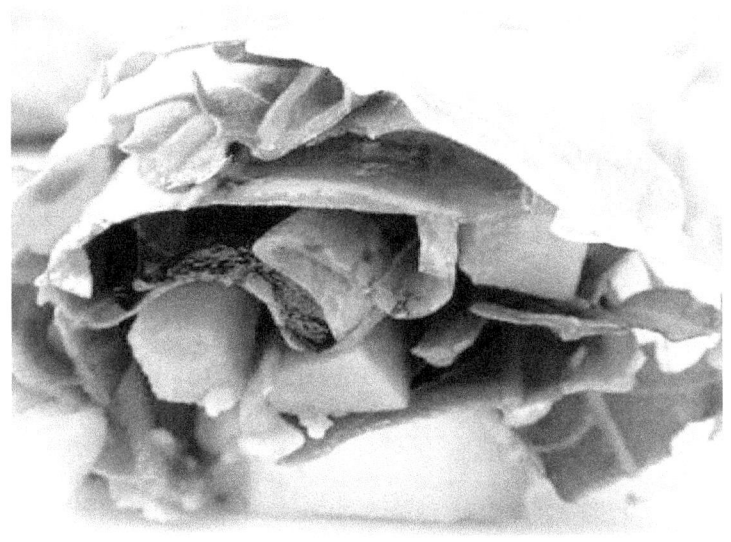

Yields 5 Servings

Ingredients

5 rice papers

A handful of spinach)

1 avocado

A handful arugula

1 carrot

5-10 leaves basil

5 olives (you can use black or green)

Optional: additional herbs

Directions

Begin by peeling the avocado and carrot and then cut them (together with the olives) into strips. Chop the spinach, basil and arugula.

Now make the rice papers soft. To do this, add warm water to a deep, round plate that's larger than the rice papers. You can use a baking tray filled with warm water and immerse the rice paper into the water for about 5 seconds. Don't let the rice paper get too soft or be too hard as that would break it. So just keep it in the water for five seconds, making sure the entire surface is covered with water; take it out and everything should be okay.

Place the doused rice paper on a plate and begin arranging the vegetables in the middle of the paper —in proportions- a little arugula, some spinach, some carrot, some basil, olives and avocado. You don't want to overfill the paper as that would make it hard to close the rolls (which would make it a rice paper mess).

Once you have everything in place in the middle, start rolling the rice paper carefully into a spring roll.

Repeat the process based on the size of your ingredients but don't soak the rice paper in advance as it will fall apart.

Chickpea Scramble Lettuce Wraps

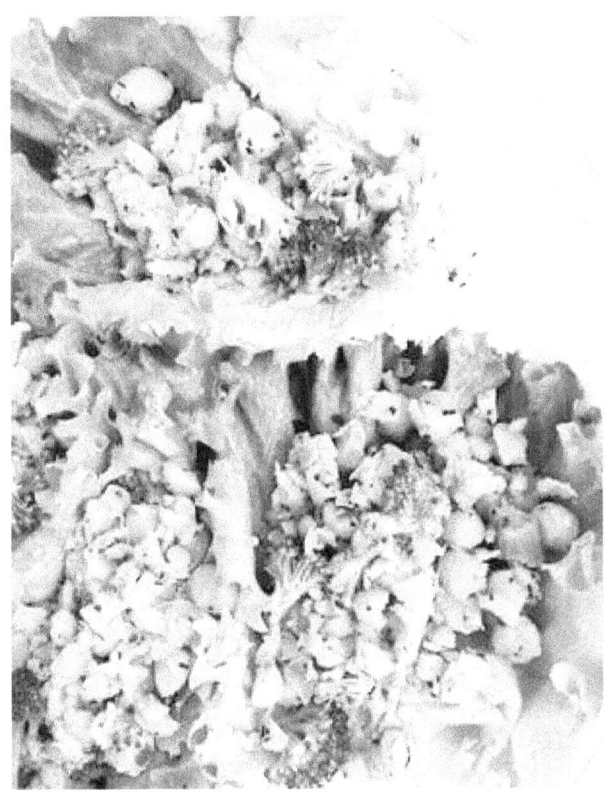

Yields 3-4 Wraps

Ingredients

1 1/2 cups chickpeas, canned

3 broccoli florets, chopped

1/3 teaspoon coriander

1 tablespoon olive oil

1/2 onion (small) or 1 scallion, chopped

1/2 teaspoon mint, dried

1/4 teaspoon chili flakes

<u>Topping or salad</u>

1/2 avocado, ripe

4 olives, chopped

4-5 lettuce leaves, washed

1 tablespoon lemon juice

5 or 6 basil leaves, chopped

Directions

Add the olive oil to a non-stick pan and then cook at medium high heat.

Press the chickpeas using a spatula and mash them as they cook. You can also use a food processor to do this (or just mash the chickpeas ahead). Just make sure the chickpeas are not too mashed-only a little bit to make them look like scrambled eggs.

When you finish mashing —most likely after 2 minutes, add the coriander, chili, mint and onion while stirring.

Add the broccoli and cover with a lid for 1-2 minutes such that the broccoli cooks up only slightly.

Turn the heat off then add the salt to taste, if needed.

Mash the avocado with the basil, chopped olives, lemon juice and some cherry tomatoes (if you have any, though this is not necessary).

To assemble the wraps, fill a lettuce leaf using 2-3 tablespoons chickpea scramble and top with the sauce.

You can sprinkle a little black pepper and flaxseed.

Serve and enjoy!

Alkaline Dinner Recipes

Kale Caesar Salad

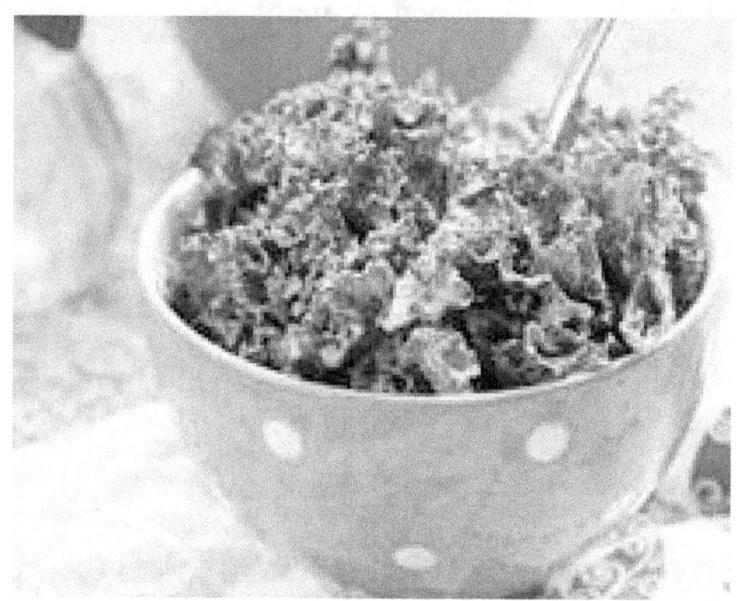

Yields 3 Servings

Ingredients

1 very large bunch of curly Kale

1/3 cup almond nuts, raw

1/2 teaspoon smoked paprika

1 1/4 filtered water

1/2 teaspoon sea salt

1 cup sunflower seeds (you can save a few to garnish if you desire)

1/8 teaspoon chipotle powder- you can adjust to your liking

2 garlic cloves

1 1/2 teaspoon agave syrup

Directions

Wash the kale leaves and pat them. Remove the middle membrane just up to where it starts thinning out making sure to tear the kale leaf into small, bite size pieces.

Add them to a large bowl and measure the rest of the ingredients into a blender and process until the mixture is creamy and smooth.

Next, pour half of the mixture nicely over the kale leaves.

Use your hands or two spoons to toss the kale to coat; add the rest of the mixture and make sure the leaves coat in folds and curls.

Let it stand for 10 minutes so that the kale leaves become tender.

Add the greens to a plate and sprinkle a few sunflower seeds, if using.

Alkaline Dinner Plate

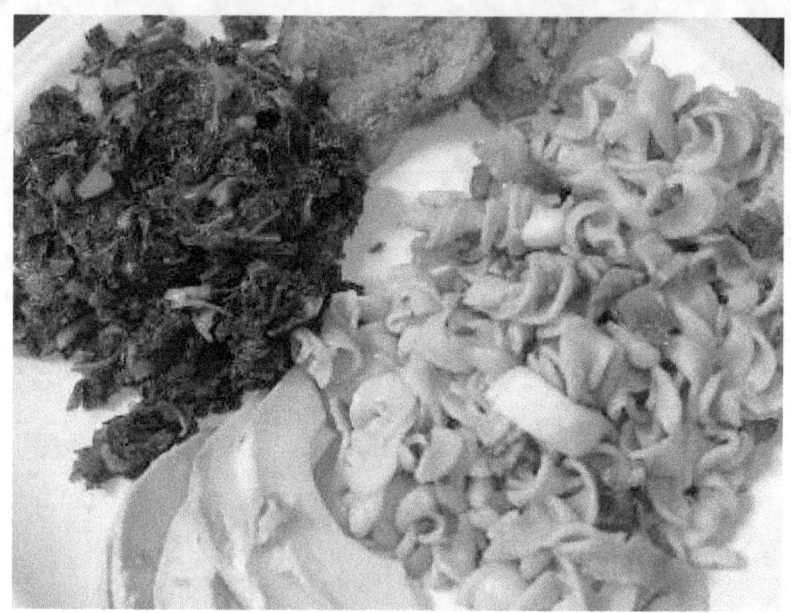

Ingredients

Yields 3 Servings

Kale Dish

1/2 cup of chopped sweet green onions, orange, yellow and red peppers

2 tablespoons of agave

Sea salt to taste

1 box Kamut pasta

1/4 cup chopped green and red onions

1/2 cup chopped yellow squash

Fried Oyster Mushrooms dish

Sea salt, cayenne pepper, onion powder and spelt flower (1/4 of habanero if preferred)

2 bundles kale greens

1/2 cup chopped red onions and 1/4 of habanero pepper (if preferred)

Pasta dish

1 cup chopped portabella mushrooms

1/4 cup chopped red and green peppers

1 teaspoon sea salt

1/2 teaspoon of grape seed oil

Avocado slices to plate if you like

Directions

Wash the kale and chop it into tiny pieces.

Coat the bottom of a pot lightly with grape seed oil.

Add the peppers and onions to the pan and sauté; and then add the kale and 2 tablespoons of agave.

Let it cook for about 30 minutes on medium heat, making sure to stir occasionally.

Let a pot of water boil, and then add grape seed oil, sea salt and add the Kamut pasta.

Get a sauce pan and sauté the peppers, onions, portabella mushrooms.

Add the cooked pasta and the veggies to the saucepan, and then add the chopped yellow squash and combine.

Rinse the oyster mushrooms lightly and season with onion powder, cayenne pepper and sea salt to your liking.

Coat with the spelt flour and fry in grape seed oil lightly.

When ready, place it on a paper towel to remove the excess oil.

Serve immediately and enjoy!

Portabella Mushrooms and Gravy

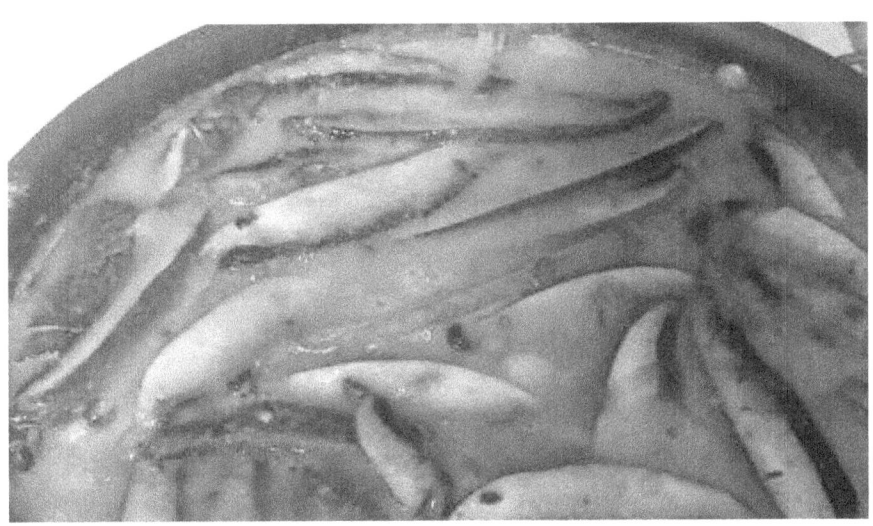

Yields 2 Servings

Ingredients

3 large portabella mushrooms

1/2 red onion

Sea salt to taste

Spelt flour

Spring water

1 long green onions

3 assorted mini organic sweet peppers

Cayenne or red bird pepper to taste

Grape seed oil

Directions

Slice the mushrooms and veggies.

Add the grape seed oil to a saucepan set over medium or high heat and add the spelt flour; stir until it becomes a soft paste.

Let the paste brown as you stir and then add water.

Keep stirring; the paste will turn into a gravy. Add more spring water until it forms a soup-like consistency.

Now add vegetables and seasonings while stirring occasionally.

Add the portabella mushrooms, stir, cover and allow the dish to simmer slowly on low medium heat.

Make sure to stir occasionally to avoid any sticking.

When ready, serve and enjoy!

Salad With Almonds and Turmeric-Dressing

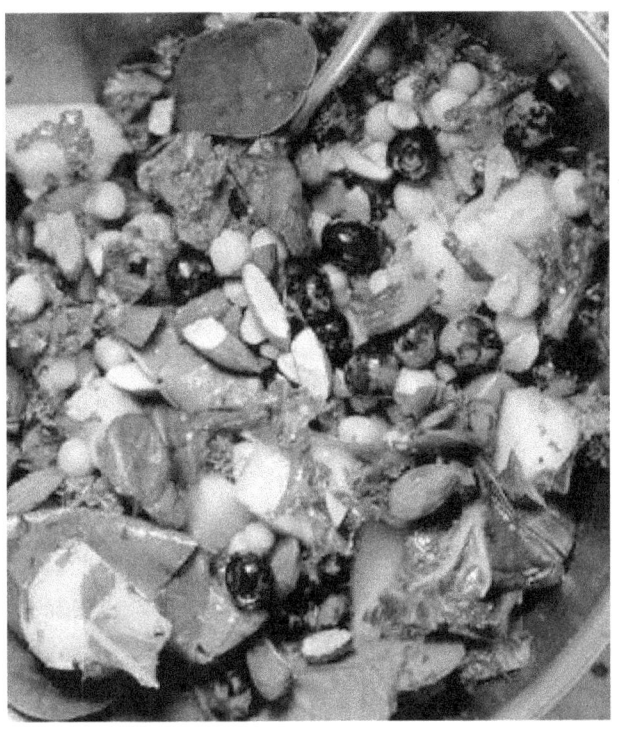

Yields 4 Servings

Ingredients

250g kale

1 bunch mint, chopped

Juice from 1 lemon

Pinch sea salt

125g fresh blueberries

2 handfuls almonds

1 bunch parsley, chopped

2 handfuls baby spinach leaves

1 teaspoon ground black pepper

3 tablespoons of cold pressed olive oil

1/2 peeled and chopped ripe pineapple

1 handful pumpkin seeds

Dressing

4 tablespoons of cold pressed olive oil

1 teaspoon fresh grated ginger

1 teaspoon agave

1 teaspoon fresh grated or ground turmeric

Juice from 1/2 lemon

Pinch sea salt and black pepper

Directions

Start by washing the kale, removing the tough inner stem and shredding it.

Place the kale into a huge mixing bowl; add some salt, pepper, olive oil and juice of 1 lemon.

Massage the kale leaves until the kale collapses, which is about 1-2 minutes.

Now add the spinach and fresh chopped mint and parsley.

Add the blueberry, pineapple, almonds, pumpkin seeds and a little turmeric dressing.

For the dressing-

Add all the dressing ingredients into a small jar and combine well until they're well integrated. Taste and adjust to your liking. Refrigerate.

Now toss through until the aromatics get distributed through the salad evenly. Divide the salad between the serving bowls and enjoy.

Baked Beans

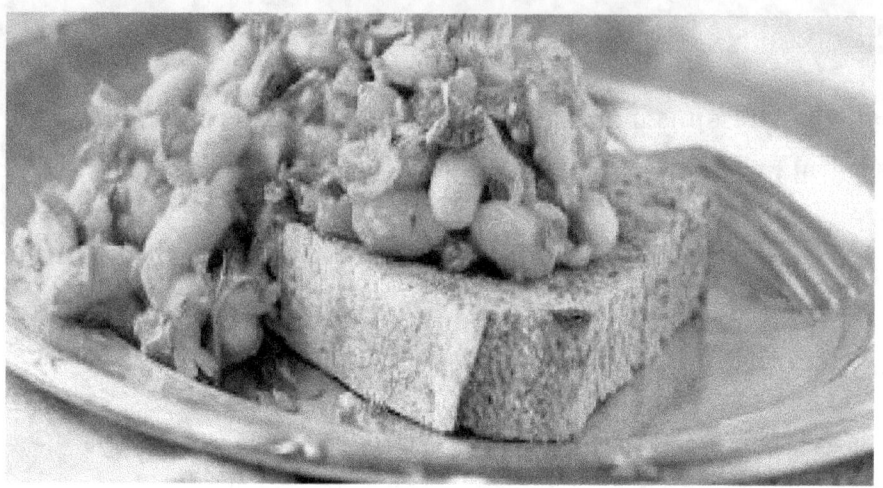

Yields 1 Serving

Ingredients

1 cup organic butter beans, rinsed well and drained

¼ white onion, diced

1 teaspoon dry mustard powder

1 teaspoon coconut oil

Sea salt to taste

1 drop liquid agave

30g avocado

2 tablespoons 100% organic tomato paste

1 garlic clove, sliced

½ teaspoon smoked paprika

1/2 cup cherry tomatoes, halved

Cracked pepper

1 cups of fresh baby spinach

Directions

Put coconut oil to a pan set over low-medium heat and sauté the garlic and onion until softened.

Add the butter beans, tomato paste and cherry tomatoes, and cook for three minutes.

Add in the seasonings and sweetener, and cook for three more minutes.

To serve, add avocado and spinach and enjoy!

Alkaline Green Energy Soup

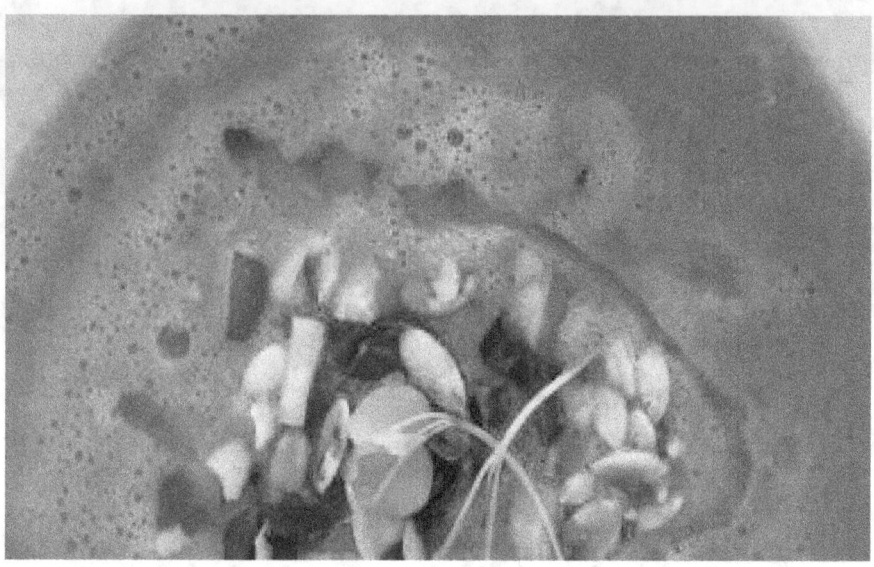

Yields 3 Servings

Ingredients

4 cups of vegetable stock (you can also can use ½ cup of almond milk or coconut to make it richer)

1 cup kale

1 cup parsley

1.5 inches fresh ginger

4 cloves garlic

1 teaspoon Himalayan sea salt

1 cup spinach

1 cup arugula

1 cup chickpeas

1 red onion

2 tablespoons turmeric

Garnish:

Pepper, to taste.

Himalayan sea salt

Greens

Extra virgin olive oil

½ of lemon for each cup of soup

¼ cup sprouted pumpkin seeds

Directions

Add all the ingredients to a large pot and cook on low or medium heat for about 20 minutes.

Transfer everything to a blender and process for a couple of seconds.

To garnish, add juice from ½ lemon, the greens, sprouted pumpkin seeds, sea salt and olive oil.

Enjoy!

Butternut Squash Quinoa Casserole

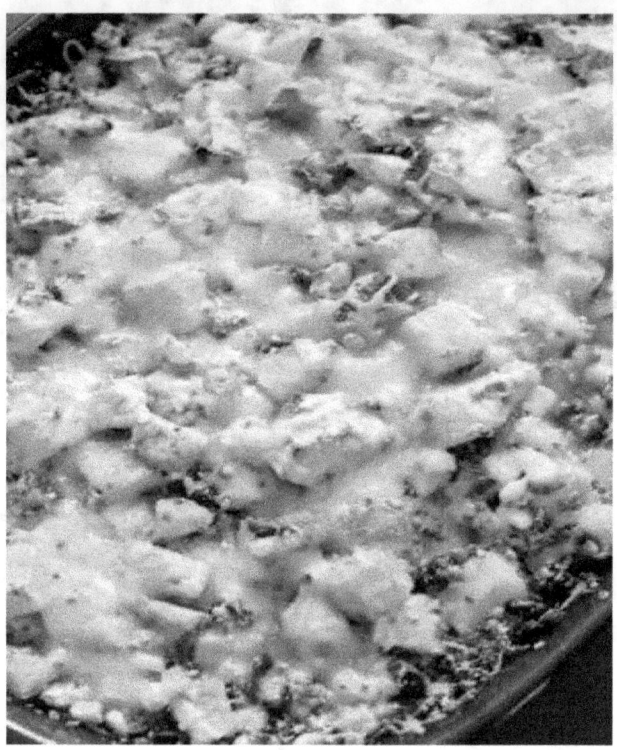

Yields 8 Servings

Ingredients

1 tablespoon of olive oil

1 cup uncooked quinoa and 2 cups water (makes 3 cups when cooked)

1 15-ounce can black beans (a bit more than one cup), drained and rinsed

1 lime, juiced

1 tomato, chopped

2 cups non-dairy cheese

6 cups cubed butternut squash

2 cups corn

1 tablespoon cumin

Salt and pepper, to taste

1 avocado, diced

Salsa or hot sauce, optional

Directions

Preheat your oven to 400 degrees F.

Roast the butternut squash with olive oil in the oven set at 400 degrees F. for 15 minutes. You can also use the stovetop (cook for 10 – 12 minutes at medium-high heat).

In the meantime, prepare the quinoa. Simply add the quinoa and water to a sauce pan and bring to a boil. Lower the heat to low and simmer until most of the water becomes absorbed- that should take about 15 minutes.

Add the cooked quinoa and squash to a large casserole dish (should be not less than 9x13) along with black beans and corn.

Add in some lime juice, cumin, pepper and salt and mix properly.

Add the avocado and tomato (though you may want to wait until after the dish bakes to add the avocado).

Top with cheese and bake for 10-15 minutes, or until the cheese melts.

Vegetable Stroganoff

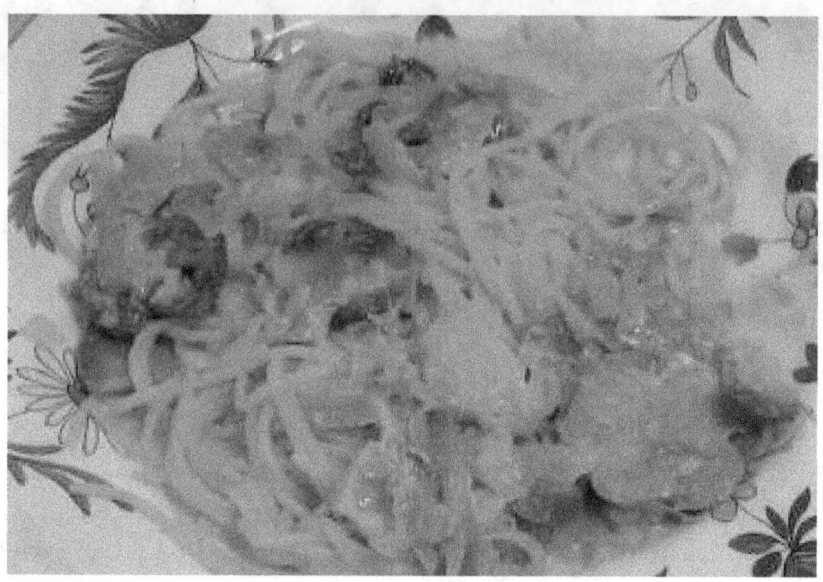

Yields 4 Servings

Ingredients

2 tablespoons olive oil

8 Brussels sprouts, sliced into quarters

1 onion, chopped

1 teaspoon sea salt

1 teaspoon dried mustard

2 tablespoons sour cream

I box of spelt pasta

2 large artichoke hearts, trimmed down to the heart with the chokes removed and sliced (Alternatively, you can use frozen or jar hearts)

1 Leek, chopped

6 ounce- box of sliced mushrooms

Pepper to taste

1 ½ cups vegetable stock (reserve ½ cup for later)

½ cup chopped parsley

Directions

Add the olive oil to a large skillet and heat; add the onions then cook them for five minutes.

Add the mushrooms and the leek and cook for 2 more minutes.

Next, add the Brussels sprouts, artichoke, pepper and salt.

Add the dried mustard while stirring and then finish by adding one cup of the vegetable stock.

Cover the dish and cook for 10-15 minutes, or until the vegetables are tender. Just make sure to check after five minutes, and add the reserved stock.

When everything is done, add the sour cream while stirring.

Add the parsley as topping and serve alongside spelt pasta.

Stuffed Zucchini

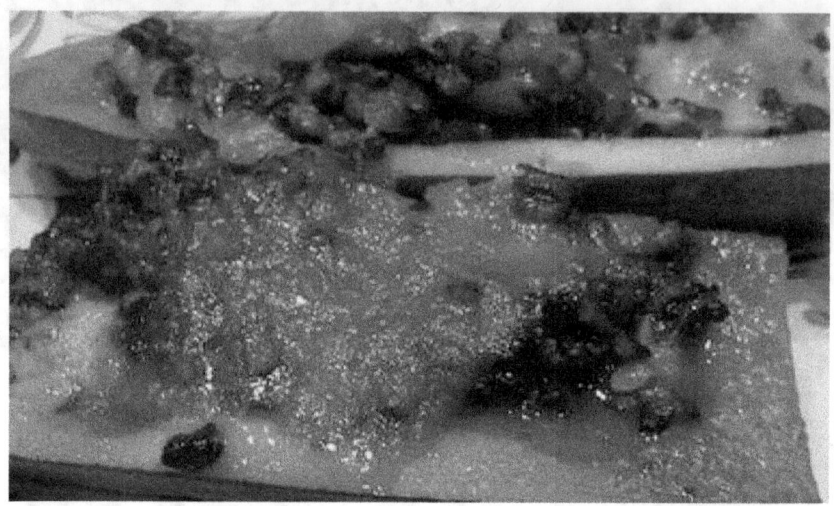

Yields 3 Servings

Ingredients

2 medium-large zucchini

2 ½ cups water

1 onion, sliced thinly

2 tablespoon olive oil

1 cup marinara sauce

1 cup japonica rice (see note about using cauliflower rice)

¼ teaspoon sea salt

1 clove garlic finely minced

Salt and pepper

Ingredients

Preheat your oven to 350 degrees F.

Add salt to the water and bring to a boil, and the cook the rice for 45 minutes- you can also use a rice cooker to cook the rice.

Add the olive oil to a large skillet, heat and add the onion; cook for ten minutes and then add the garlic.

Scoop out the flesh of the zucchini with a melon ball spoon; you'll be left with four zucchini boats that are ready for filling and a pile of zucchini balls.

Cut the zucchini balls in quarters and add the onions.

Season with pepper and salt, to taste.

When you confirm that the rice is ready, scoop one cup into the zucchini and onions mixture. Combine and adjust the seasonings if necessary.

Now combine by adding the tomato marinara at the bottom of your baking dish.

Put the zucchini boats into a casserole and fill each piece with the rice-onion mixture.

Cover using tin foil and bake for a period of 45 minutes to one hour at 350 degrees.

Serve and enjoy!

Note: Any type of rice is slightly acidic so it's most prudent to consume it as sparingly and infrequently as possible. When you decide to take it though, this right here is your recipe! If you want to make it completely alkaline, use cauliflower rice instead. To cook the cauliflower rice, sauté the cauliflower rice using 1 tablespoon of olive oil inside a skillet then cover with a lid to allow the cauliflower to steam and become a lot more tender. Cook it for 5-8 minutes before seasoning with salt and pepper.

Cauliflower Gnocchi

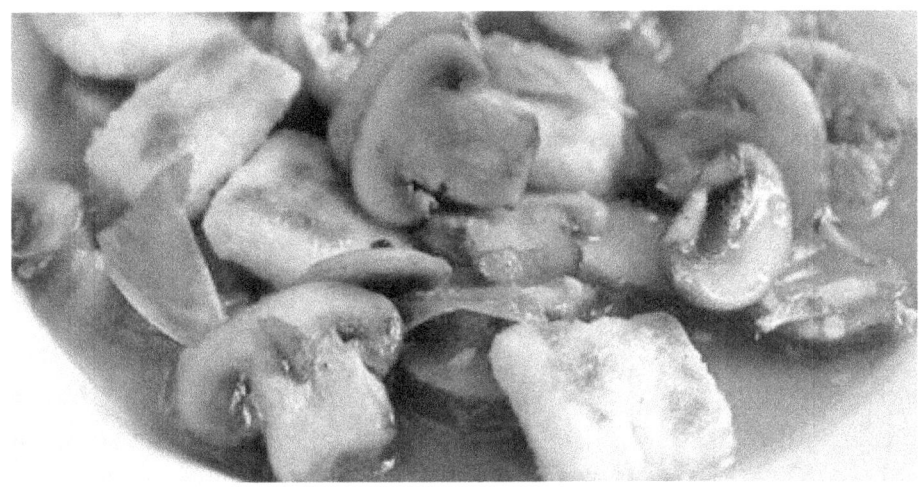

Yields 4 Servings

Ingredients

1 head of cauliflower, steamed or boiled until very tender

1 cup spelt flour- or enough to make soft dough

1 clove garlic, finely chopped

1 tablespoon olive or coconut oil to fry

<u>The Ragout</u>

1 tin whole tomatoes

½ onion, finely sliced

2 finely sliced garlic cloves

300 ml vegetable stock

Fresh basil, to serve

4 courgettes, thickly sliced

1 tablespoon olive or coconut oil

6 thickly sliced black mushrooms

1 teaspoon date sugar, salt and pepper to taste

Directions

Add the garlic and cauliflower to a food processor or blender and process until fine and smooth. You can add some water if you want to have a smooth paste.

Add the flour and salt, ¼ cup at a time, and continue processing until you have soft dough. Again, add some more water as necessary.

Turn it out on a clean, floured surface and knead it for a little while, until the dough becomes soft and smooth.

Cut the dough into 4 pieces then take one piece and cover the other three using a damp tea towel.

Next, roll the dough into a 3 cm (-or so) rope, and then cut it into pieces.

Using a fork, press each piece down and set aside; repeat the process with the rest of the dough.

Add the oil to a non-stick pan or pot then heat and fry the gnocchi until both sides brown lightly.

For the ragout, add the coconut oil to a non-stick pot set over medium heat and then fry the garlic, onion, courgettes and mushrooms until they start to color and soften.

Next, add the tomatoes, sugar and vegetable stock, reduce the heat to medium and let it simmer gently for 15 minutes, or until the vegetables become tender. Season to taste.

To serve, top the ragout with the warm cauliflower gnocchi and a few basil leaves.

Enjoy!

Grilled Courgette Salad

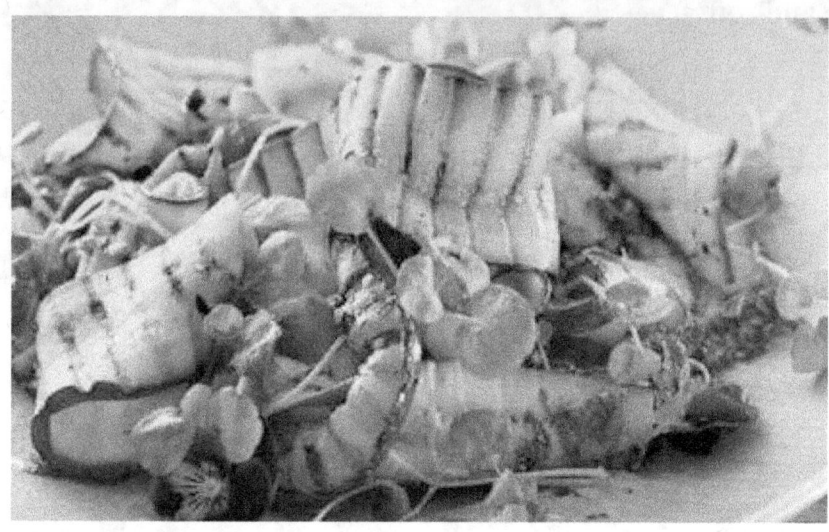

Yields 2 Servings

Ingredients

6 courgettes

Sea salt

80g watercress

<u>Dressing</u>

Zest and juice of 1/2 lemon

15g fresh mint leaves

Salt pepper

1 red chili

6 tablespoons extra-virgin olive oil

Directions

Wash the watercress and courgettes.

Then slice the courgettes lengthwise and thinly such that you have flat strips.

Add a sprinkle of sea salt and allow them to soften a bit as their water gets extracted by the salt.

To make the dressing, wash the chili, lemon and mint leaves; remove the chili seeds and chop it into fine pieces. Shred the leaves.

Now add the chili, lemon zest, mint, olive oil and the lemon juice/zest to a bowl and whisk.

Season the mixture with pepper and salt.

Put the watercress in a serving dish.

The barbecue-

Prepare your barbecue for direct heat, which should be roughly 220 degrees C.

Put the courgette strips on the grate, close the lid and grill each side for 3-4 minutes; some nice, dark grill marks should form; take them off when ready and let them cool.

Put the courgettes on the watercress and pour the dressing over them.

Enjoy!

Salad With Avocado Dressing

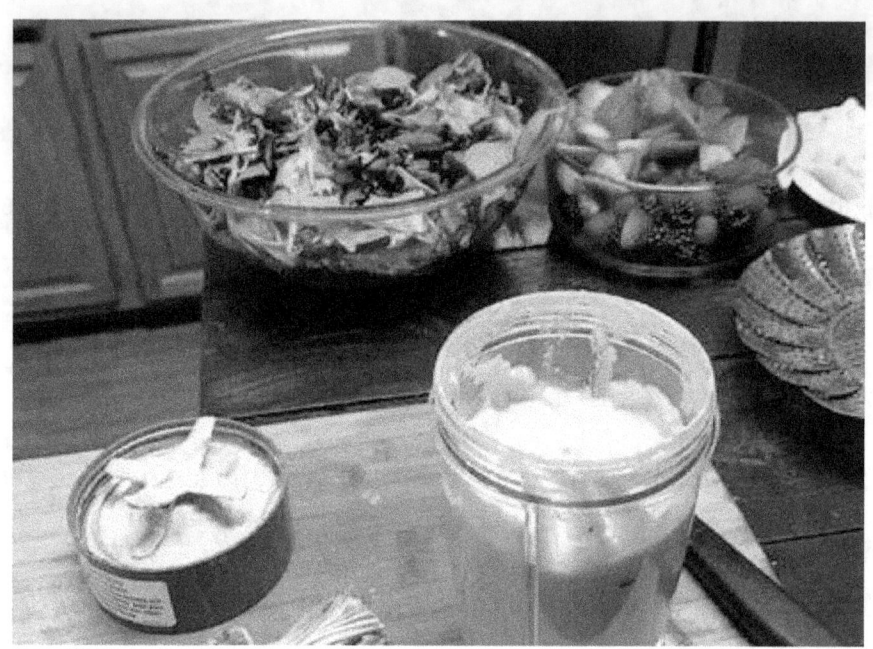

Yields 4 Servings

Ingredients

<u>The salad</u>

1 head cauliflower, cut into florets

1/2 small red onion, cut into 4 pieces

1 bunch kale, stems removed and shredded

1/4 cup raw sunflower seeds

1/2 head red cabbage, cut into 8 pieces

2 medium carrots, peeled

1 bunch cilantro -or flat-leaf parsley, finely chopped

1/4 cup raw shelled hemp seeds

The dressing

2 medium avocados, mashed

1 medium lemon, juiced, plus more to taste

1 tablespoon finely chopped cilantro

Celtic sea salt to taste

1/4 cup apple cider vinegar

1 clove garlic, minced

1 tablespoon minced fresh ginger

Freshly ground black pepper to taste

Directions

Fit your food processor with the s-blade and proceed to rice your cauliflower: add the florets to the food processor and process until you get a couscous consistency.

After that, add the onion and red cabbage to the food processor and pulse until it is finely chopped.

Now fit the dicing disc into the processor if you have one and dice the carrots (you can also dice them with your hands using a knife).

Add the processed cabbage, onion, cauliflower and carrot to a large bowl and toss along with cilantro, chopped kale, sunflower seeds and raisins (if you're using them).

Place in the fridge to cool as you prepare the dressing.

For the dressing, just add all the salad ingredients to a bowl and whisk.

Serve by tossing the dressing through the salad; add some lemon juice, pepper and salt to taste.

Enjoy immediately.

Shiitake Cauliflower Fried Rice

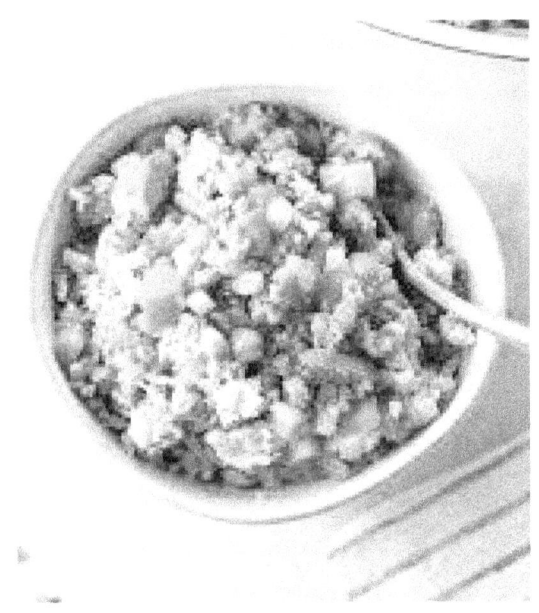

Yields 4 Servings

Ingredients

1 large head cauliflower

2 tablespoons toasted sesame oil

2 tablespoons minced fresh ginger

6 green onions, finely chopped (the white and green parts)

2 + ½ tablespoons of wheat-free tamari

2 + ½ teaspoons fresh lime juice

2 tablespoons grape seed oil

1 small green chili, ribbed, seeded, and minced

4 teaspoons minced garlic (4 cloves)

4 cups of shiitake mushrooms, finely chopped

1 finely chopped bunch of cilantro

Celtic sea salt to taste

Directions

Start by chopping the cauliflower into florets and throw away the leaves as well as the tough middle core.

Add the cauliflower pieces to a food processor (with an S-blade) and process for a few seconds, until you get a rice-like consistency. In the end, you should be having 5 or 6 cups of cauliflower rice.

Add the oil to a deep skillet or wok and heat the oil on medium-high heat, and sauté the chili, garlic, mushrooms, green onions and ginger with ¼ teaspoon of salt for 5 or so minutes, until soft and properly combined.

Add the cauliflower rice and tamari, and sauté for five more minutes, until everything is soft.

Add the lime juice, cilantro and the rest of the salt while stirring, and adjust the flavors to taste.

Soba Noodles with Turmeric Thai Sauce

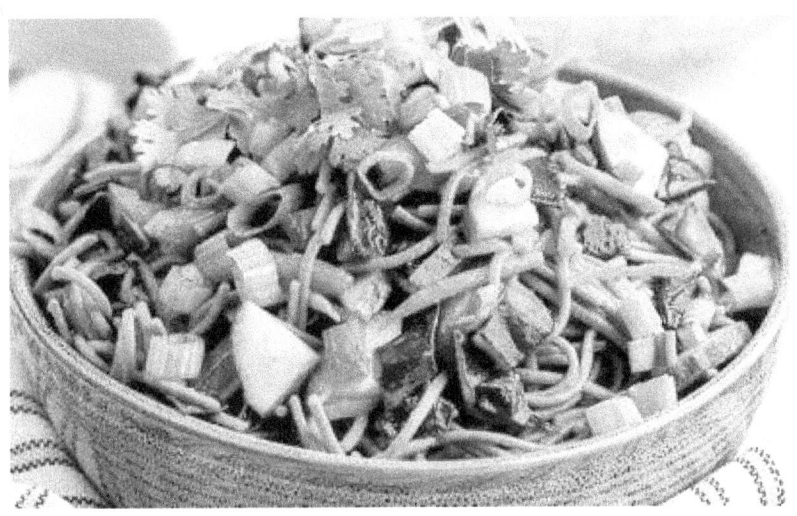

Yields 5 Servings

Ingredients

1 package buckwheat soba noodles

1 cup red bell pepper, thinly sliced

½ cup red cabbage, thinly sliced

1 cucumber, chopped

1 cup carrots, shredded

1 cup green bell pepper, thinly sliced

½ cup green onions, chopped

1/3 cup cilantro

Dressing

2 tablespoons coconut aminos

1 teaspoon sesame oil

2 tablespoons hot water

½ teaspoon ground turmeric

1 teaspoon black pepper

1 teaspoon agave syrup

1 tablespoon nut butter of choice

½ teaspoon ground ginger

½ teaspoon garlic powder

Directions

Mix the dressing ingredients and set aside.

Cook the buckwheat noodles following the instructions on the package and set aside.

Add the noodles to a bowl along with the chopped vegetables.

Add the dressing and combine properly.

Top with sliced green onions and serve.

Enjoy!

Spring Vegetable Quinoa Bowl

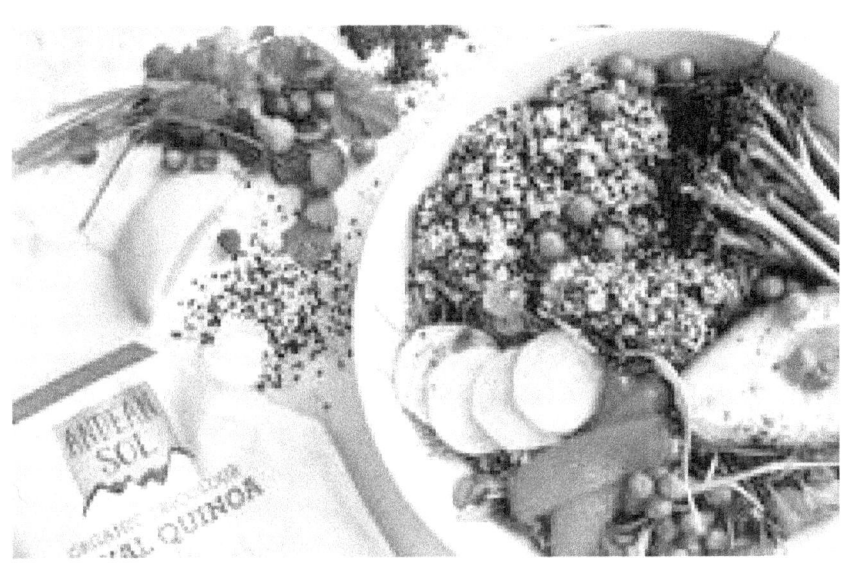

Yields 2 Servings

Ingredients

150g quinoa

45g watercress

120g purple sprouting broccoli

1 tin chickpeas, drained and rinsed

45g rocket

2 beetroots, sliced

1 red pepper, sliced

Optional ingredients

1 avocado, for garnish

1 handful fresh coriander, for garnish

1 tablespoon tahini, to dress

1 sprinkle chili flakes, for garnish

1 lemon, juice, for garnish

Directions

Wash all the vegetables and slice them.

Prepare the quinoa according to packet instructions.

Preheat your oven to 200 degrees C. then line a medium-sized baking tray with parchment paper and place the chickpeas and sliced vegetables on it.

Drizzle some olive oil, pepper and salt over them and bake for 20-25 minutes.

Make sure to flip after every ten minutes.

The vegetables should have a soft texture, and the chickpeas should be bit crunchy on the exterior.

Bring everything together in a large bowl and top with any desired garnishes and dressing.

Alkaline Snack/Dessert Recipes

Banana Slices

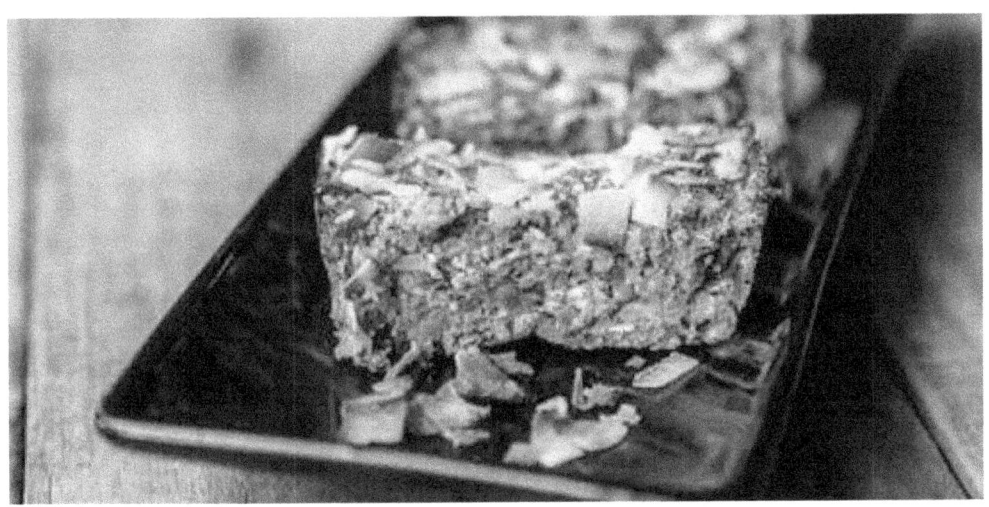

Yields 16 pieces

Ingredients

3 large ripe bananas

1/4 cup dried dates finely chopped

¼ cup slivered almonds

1/4 cup sunflower seeds

1 1/2 teaspoon vanilla extract

3 cups traditional rolled oats

1/4 cup dried apricots finely chopped

1/4 cup chia seeds

1 teaspoon ground cinnamon

1 tablespoons coconut shredded

Directions

Preheat your oven to 160 degrees C.

Grease a slice pan with a base (measuring 16cm x 25.5cm) and line it with baking paper. Extend the paper 2 cm above the edges of the pan.

Add the banana until smooth, and then add the rest of the ingredients and combine well to give you a nicely blended mixture (a food processor is best used here).

When the mixture is well integrated, add it to the pan you prepared and press it into the pan evenly; top with shredded coconut.

Bake for 30 to 35 minutes until golden and then let it cool completely. Cut it into small bars and serve.

Enjoy!

Cherry and Quinoa Truffles

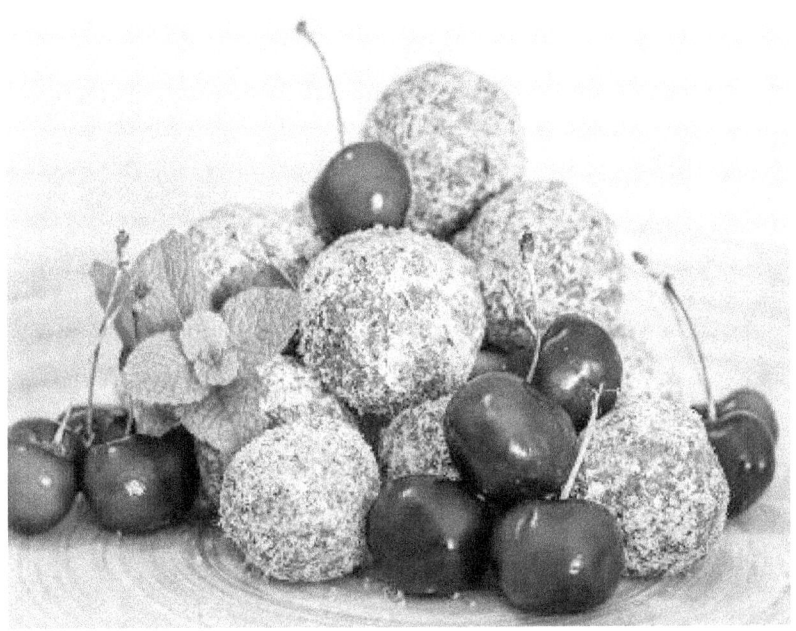

Yields 15 Balls (3 Servings)

Ingredients

100g white quinoa, cooked & cooled as per packet

100g cherries, frozen or fresh, pitted

100g raw cashews, soaked for 4 hours, drained

75g coconut, desiccated

40g agave

50g coconut flour

Directions

Add all the ingredients to a food processor or blender except some coconut (50g) and process until well integrated, and until you have dough that you can roll into balls.

Roll the dough into balls and toss it lightly in the remaining coconut.

You can store the balls in a fridge for one week or in the freezer for two months

Enjoy!

Coconut Chia Cream Pots

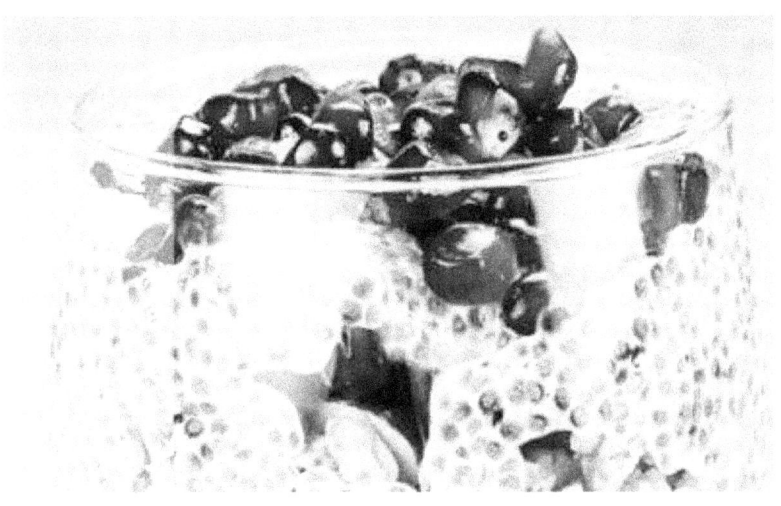

Yields 4 Servings

Ingredients

1 cup of (organic) coconut milk

1 date

1 tablespoon of flax meal or 1 tablespoon of ground flax seeds

1/2 teaspoon of vanilla extract

1/4 cup of chia seeds

1 cup of coconut yoghurt

1 teaspoon of sesame seeds

<u>Toppings</u>

1 handful of blueberries

1 teaspoon of ground cinnamon

1 handful of mixed nuts (such as almonds, brazil nuts, macadamia and pistachios)

1 fig

Directions

Blend the coconut milk with the date to add a touch of sweetness to the milk.

Now add the coconut milk to a large bowl, along with the ground flax, sesame seeds, chia seeds and vanilla.

Put the mixture in the fridge for 20-30 minutes, until the chia expands.

Fill a little glass with a layer of coconut yoghurt and then another layer of the chia mix and small additional layer of coconut yoghurt.

Top with anything you like and enjoy!

Chocolate Cereal Candy Bar Treat

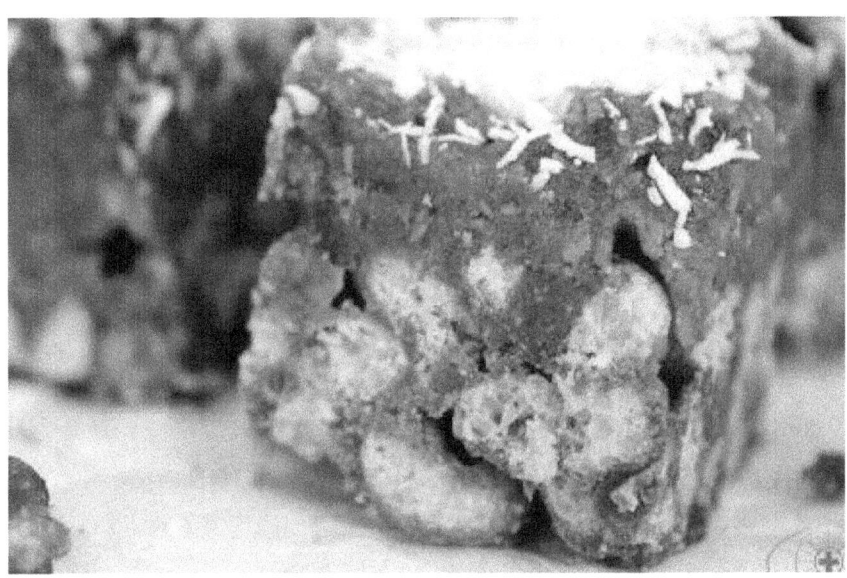

Yields 1 Candy Bar

Ingredients

1 cup chocolate almond butter

2 cups desired alkaline cereal (such as kamut cereal)

Toppings

Unsweetened coconut flakes

1/2 cup blended dates

Directions

Start by preparing the chocolate almond butter. Add the almond butter and cereal to a large mixing bowl and stir until the cereal is well integrated.

Add the mixture to a baking sheet lined with parchment paper and place it in the freezer so that it sets quickly.

Add soft pitted dates to a food processor and blend to a paste. Spread it over the cereal candy when it hardens.

Add the coconut flakes as topping.

Let the candy bar harden in the freezer and then store it in the refrigerator- in a covered dish.

Roasted Cinnamon Chickpeas

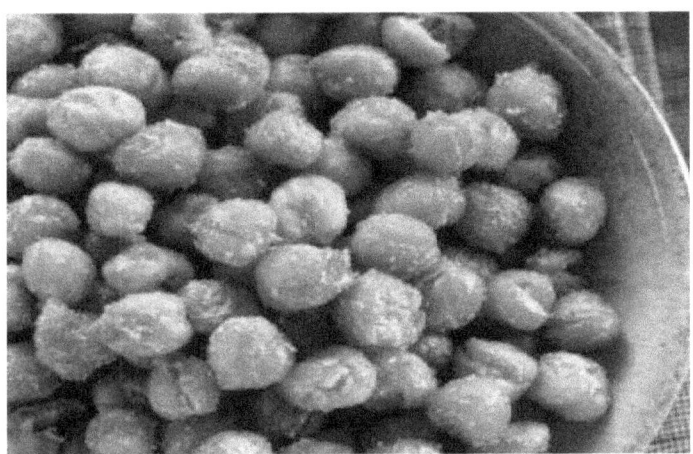

Yields 2 Servings

Ingredients

1 carton of already in water organic chickpeas

2 tablespoons of organic coconut oil

2 tablespoons of cinnamon powder

Directions

Add the melted coconut oil to a bowl of rinsed chickpeas.

Add the cinnamon and combine.

Line a baking tray with a non-stick parchment paper and then add the mixture to it.

Roast until the exterior becomes slightly crispy. This should take about half an hour at 180 degrees C.

Alkaline Avocado Sandwich

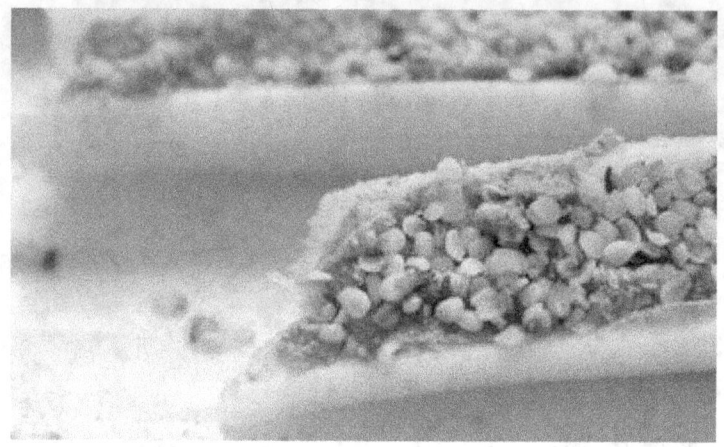

Yields 1 Serving

Ingredients

<u>The baguette</u>

200g sunflower seeds

2 tablespoons extra virgin cold-pressed olive oil

200g flax seeds

Your favorite alkaline spices

<u>The spread</u>

1 ripe avocado

2 tablespoons extra virgin cold-pressed olive oil

1 clove of garlic

Sea salt and pepper to taste

Directions

As you start, keep it in mind that this snack is best made a day before you eat it.

Prepare the cauliflower seeds and flax seeds by soaking (the cauliflower seeds) and grinding (the flax seeds) them. Mix them with spices, if using, and oil and create little slices of bread.

Store in a food dehydrator set at 104 degrees F- overnight

To make the spread, mix the oil, avocado and garlic together and add pepper and salt to taste.

Enjoy!

Vanilla Bean Ice Cream

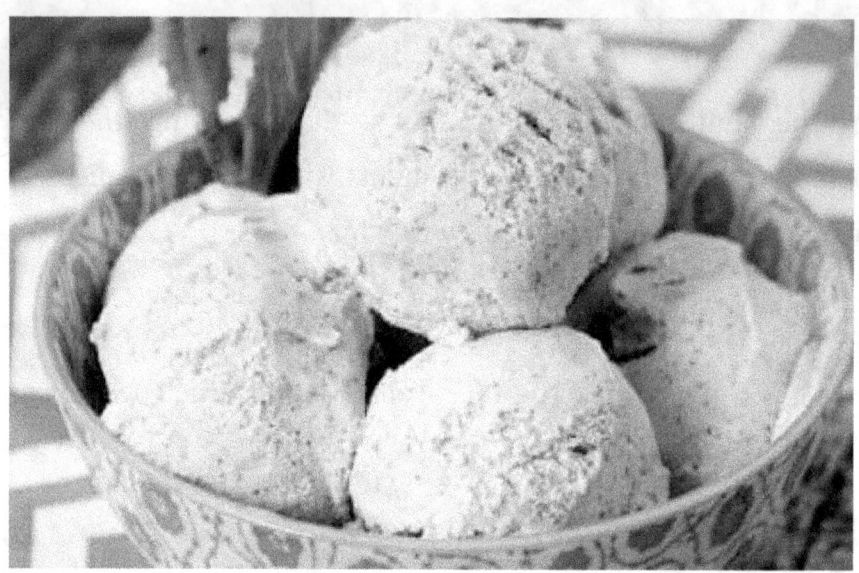

Yields 3 Servings

Ingredients

2 13.5-ounce cans full-fat organic coconut milk

2 teaspoons organic vanilla extract

1 pinch Himalayan pink salt

1/2 cup organic granular sweetener

1 teaspoon organic vanilla bean powder

Sweetener

Directions

Add everything to a blender and process until well integrated.

Pour the mixture into an ice-cream machine and follow the machine instructions to make the ice-cream.

When the ice-cream is done, dig in and enjoy it as a soft serve ice.

Alternatively, you can add the mixture to a freezer-safe container and freeze it, covered, for a few hours, until the mixture becomes firm to the usual consistency of ice-cream.

Dig in and enjoy!

Raw Walnut Fudge

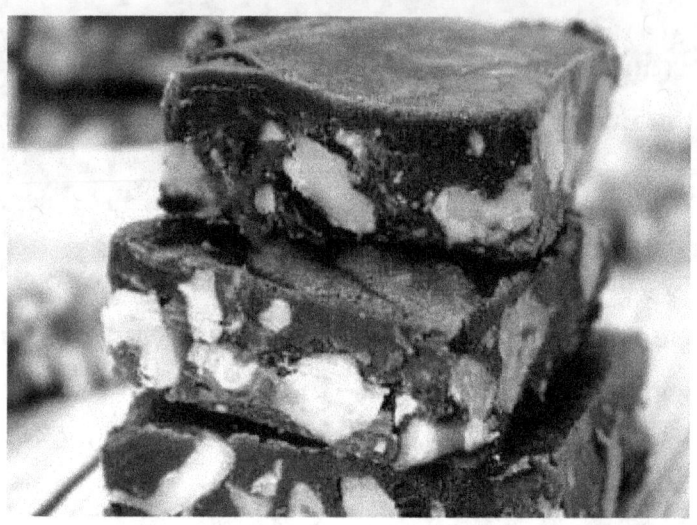

Yields 8 Fudges

Ingredients

1 cup organic coconut oil (melted/liquid)

1/4 cup agave syrup

1/4 cup organic walnuts (chopped)

Organic date nectar

1/4 cup organic raw cacao powder

1/4 cup organic almond butter

1 teaspoon organic vanilla bean powder

Directions

Add everything to a bowl and stir properly until smooth and well integrated.

Spread the mixture evenly in a bread pan.

Place it in the freezer for roughly 30- 60 minutes, or until the mixture hardens.

Pour it into an airtight container and store in the freezer until it's ready to serve.

Enjoy!

Note: When you leave it out at room temperature, it will soften and lose its shape.

Tropical Papaya Boats

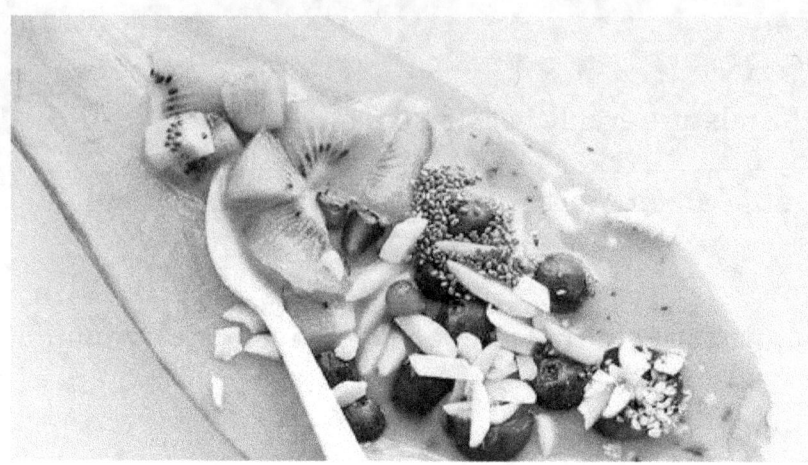

Yields 1 Serving

Ingredients

1 medium kiwi fruit (without skin, chopped)

1/4 cup blueberries

1 tablespoon chia seeds

1/2 tablespoon hulled hemp seeds, shelled

1/2 cup pitted sweet cherry, raw (halved)

2 tablespoons slivered almonds

2 bananas, ripe and frozen

1 tablespoon granola

Almond milk

1 medium papaya

Directions

Make banana ice cream by adding two ripe, sliced, frozen bananas to a food processor or blender and process on low speed until you get a creamy ice consistency. Scrape down the container's side to remove as much of the banana as possible (add some almond milk if needed).

Now assemble the cantaloupe or papaya boats by filling the hollow centers with the banana ice-cream and/or any other ingredient you desire such as the berries, seeds and nuts.

Enjoy immediately!

Cheesy Dill Kale Chips

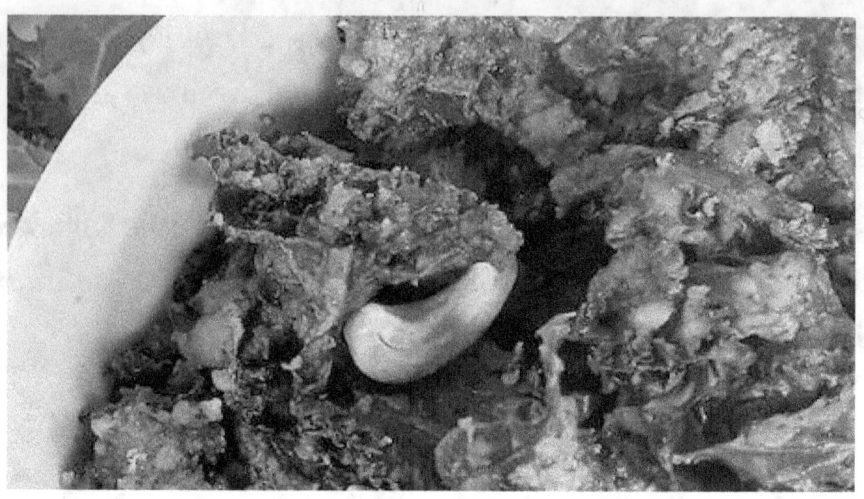

Serves 8

Ingredients

1 bunch kale (stems removed and cut into bite sized pieces or 'chips')

1/3 cup nutritional yeast

1/2 medium lemon (juiced)

1 1/2 tablespoons dill, fresh

1/2 teaspoon onion powder

1/4 cup water (add a few extra tablespoons to add until desired consistency is reached)

1 cup cashew nuts, raw (soaked in water for not less than 30 minutes beforehand and drained)

4 tablespoons extra-virgin olive oil

1 teaspoon apple cider

1/2 teaspoon garlic powder

1 tablespoon salt

1 teaspoon black pepper

Directions

Preheat oven to 275 degrees F and then wash the kale well.

Drizzle "cheese sauce" (directions below) over it evenly, making sure it is well coated.

Then spread your chips evenly on a parchment paper lined baking sheet to form a neat layer.

Place in the oven and bake for 25-35 minutes. Make sure to flip halfway.

Cheese sauce preparation

Add all the ingredients apart from the kale to a blender. Add ¼ cup of water slowly as you pulse. Now add the water bit by bit (1 tablespoon at a time) until you get a sauce consistency. This is your cheese sauce.

2 Ingredient Banana & Coconut Cookies

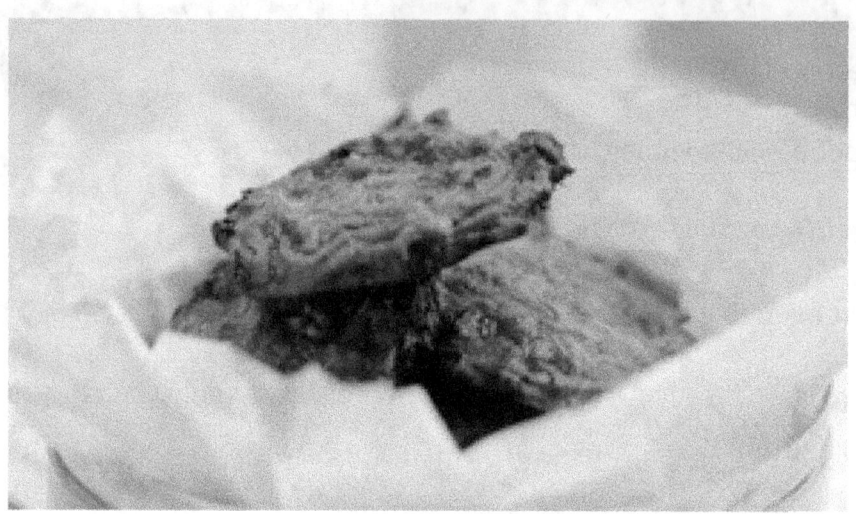

Yields 7 Pieces

Ingredients

1 large, ripe banana

3⁄4 cup shredded coconut

Directions

Preheat your oven to 350 degrees F and then line a baking tray with a sheet of baking paper.

Add the coconut to a pan set over medium heat and toast until it browns a bit.

Remove from the heat and add it to a blender; add the banana and blend until the coconut is fine and the mixture is desirable.

Add the mixture to discs spaced evenly on the baking tray. You can spoon the mixture into the tray if it is runny.

Bake for about 25 minutes, until golden.

Enjoy!

Vegan Banana Nice-cream

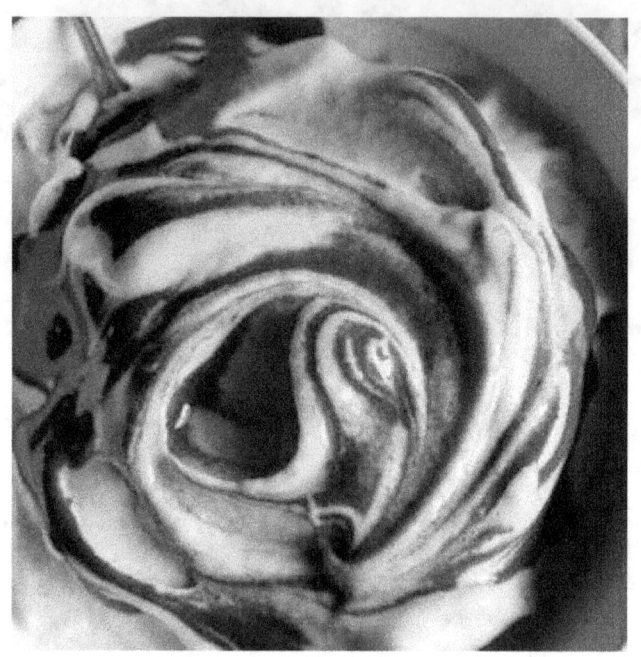

Yields 2 Servings

Ingredients

4 peeled, frozen bananas

1 cup almond milk (or water)

1 teaspoon vanilla powder

Chocolate drizzle

1 teaspoon cacao powder

1 tablespoon alkaline sweetener

1 teaspoon water

Directions

Cut the bananas into chunks each measuring 1 inch and add them to a blender.

Then add the almond milk or water, and the vanilla and blend until the mixture's consistency is like that of soft serve ice cream. Before you begin, it might not seem like you'll reach this stage but it all happens fast- all of a sudden you have a blender full of a thick, creamy ice cream!

Add this to a bowl.

For the chocolate drizzle

Simply stir the chocolate drizzle ingredients together until smooth. The cacao will take a second to combine with the liquid. Just pour it over your ice cream and enjoy. You can add anything else you desire here such as chia seeds, cinnamon, hemp seeds, berries, coconut or even berries.

Alkaline Electric Zucchini Cakes

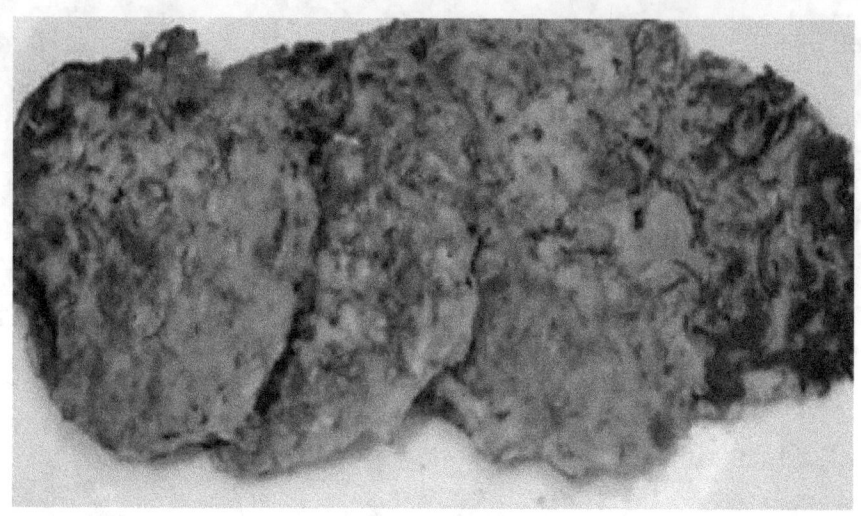

Yields 8-10 Cakes

Ingredients

2-3 zucchini

1/4 cup chopped onions

1/2 teaspoon cayenne powder

1 teaspoon sea salt

1 teaspoon parsley

Grape seed oil

1/2 cup garbanzo bean flour

1/4 cup chopped green onions

1 teaspoon onion powder

1 teaspoon oregano

1/4 cup hemp milk

Directions

Shred up the zucchini and using a strainer (or your hands), squeeze the moisture out of it.

Put it in a bowl and add the flour, onions, milk and seasonings.

Add the oil to a skillet set over medium heat and heat it. Pour the zucchini mixture into the skillet and pat it down nicely with a spatula.

Allow the cakes to cook for 3-5 minutes before you flip them on each side.

Enjoy your cakes!

Candied Walnuts & Strawberry Dressing

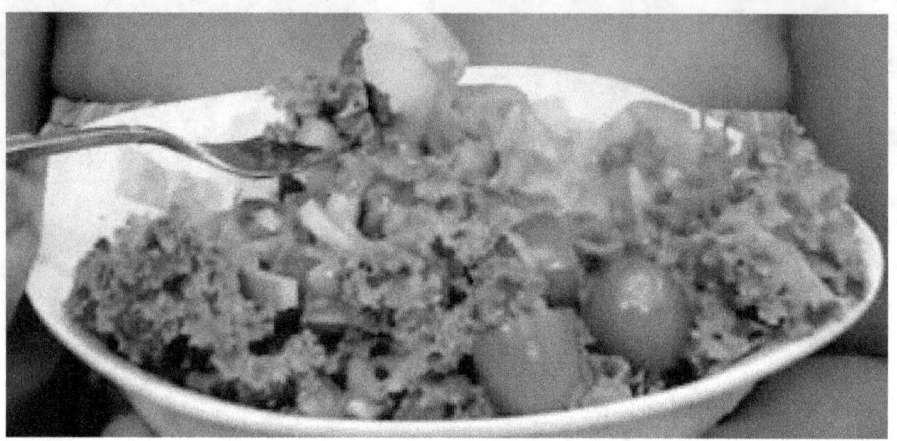

Serves 1

Ingredients

<u>Walnuts</u>

1 tablespoon raw agave nectar

1/2 cup walnuts

1/4 teaspoon sea salt

<u>Strawberry Salad Dressing</u>

1/2 cup sliced strawberries

1/2 cup grape seed oil (you can also use olive or avocado oils)

1 1/2 teaspoons lime juice

1/2 teaspoon ginger

1/4 teaspoon sea salt

2 tablespoons shallots

2 teaspoons raw agave nectar

1 teaspoon onion powder

1/4 teaspoon dill

Directions

For the walnuts-

Coat the walnuts with sea salt and agave.

Line a cookie sheet with parchment paper and place the cookies in it.

Bake for 8-10 minutes, at 325 degrees F.

Cool and enjoy- either as a snack or on your salads.

For the dressing-

Add all the ingredients to a cup or mixing bowl and mix for 30 seconds.

Enjoy!

As I have already stated, it is critical to drink lots of alkaline fluids like water, teas, juices, smoothies (I highlighted several earlier in the book) etc. You can also introduce a new twist to your alkaline foods and drinks by making herbal teas and drinks. Therefore, even if a meal may not be alkaline (remember you don't have to abandon your favorite foods – you just have to reduce them and take them 20% of the times), insist on something alkalizing like a smoothie, tea, juice, water or drink. Next, we will discuss herbs you can use to prepare various drinks and teas.

Top Alkaline Herbs

We'll now take a look at some of the best herbs that you should consider following the alkaline diet. You'll learn some of the most important details of each herb, and how to prepare it as a tea.

Let's begin.

Dill

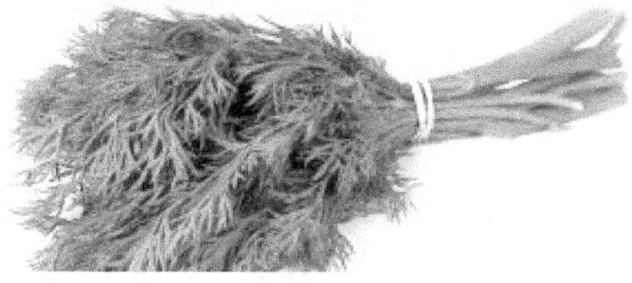

Scientific name: Anethum graveolens

Common name: Dill

Used parts: Seeds and leaves

Common medical uses:

• Boosting digestion, treating flatulence and stomach ache

• Preventing insomnia

- Improving bone health and preventing osteoporosis

- Management of diabetes

- Boosting immunity

Dill Tea

Yields 1 Serving

Ingredients

1 teaspoon dill seeds

1 cup boiling water

Directions

Using a grinder, crush the dill seeds. Bring 1 cup of water to a boil. Add one teaspoon of the crushed seeds to the boiling water and then steep (while covered) to taste.

Enjoy!

Peppermint

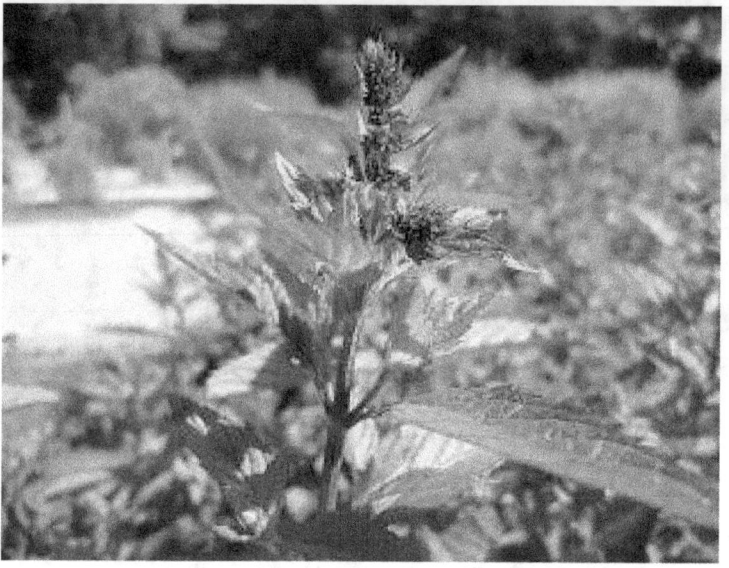

Scientific name: Mentha x piperita

Common names: Peppermint, menthol, mint

Used parts: leaves

Common medical uses:

- Improving dyspepsia

- Treating flatulence

- Easing spasms of the bile duct

- Treating gastrointestinal tract problems, biliary disorders, gastritis and intestinal colic

- Easing sinus congestion and the inflammation of the mucous membrane in the nose and throat

Peppermint Tea

Yields 2 Servings

Ingredients

2 cups water (filtered)

Optional: 2 teaspoons agave sugar or your preferred alkaline sweetener

Optional: lemon slices

15 mint leaves (fresh peppermint)

Optional: ice

Optional: lemon juice

Directions

Boil the water then add the boiling water to a cup containing the mint leaves and steep while covered for 3 – 5 minutes- you can steep longer or shorter, depending on the strength you want.

Add an alkaline sweetener if desired.

Pour the tea into mugs and garnish with slices of lemon and lemon juice to taste.

If serving iced, simply fill a tall glass with ice and pour the tea over it.

Enjoy!

Sage

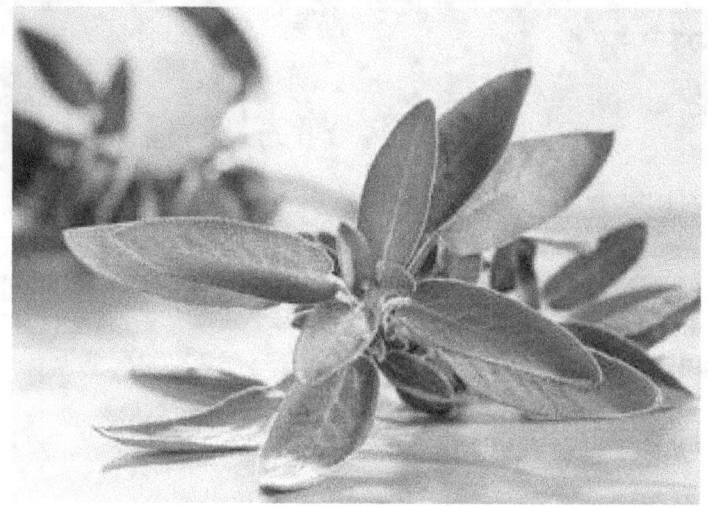

Scientific name: Salvia officinalis

Common name: sage

Used parts: leaves

Common medical uses:

- Treating and relieving digestive problems such as loss of appetite, diarrhea, heartburn, stomach pain and bloating

- Reducing excessive perspiration and saliva

- Reducing depression and memory loss

- Reducing symptoms of Alzheimer's disease

- Easing painful menstrual cramps

- Correcting excessive milk flow in nursing women

Sage Tea

Yields 1 Serving

Ingredients

1 tablespoon fresh sage leaves or 1 teaspoon dried sage

1 wedge lemon (optional)

1 cup water

Sweetener (optional)

Directions

Add the water to a pot and bring to a boil. When the water is boiling, pour it into a cup containing the sage then cover. Allow it to steep for 3-5 minutes.

Strain, as you empty the contents to a different cup.

If desired, add a sweetener and lemon, then drink. You can enjoy this beverage hot or cold.

Ginger

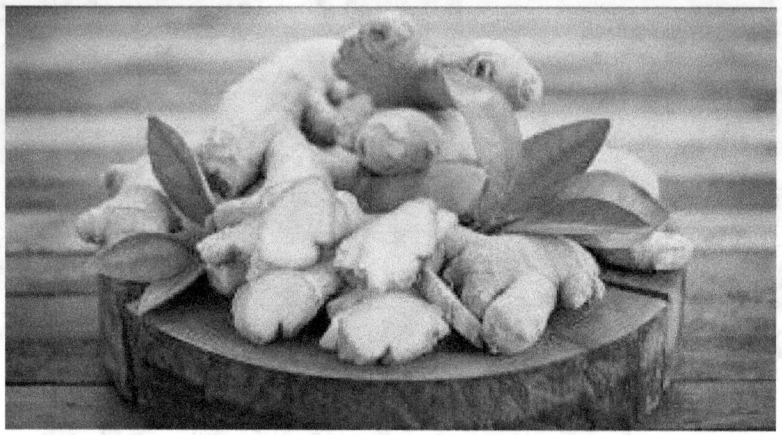

Scientific name: *Zingiber officinale*

Common name: Ginger

Used part: root

Common medical uses

- Treatment of nausea

- Easing vomiting

- Treatment of dyspepsia

- Relieving inflammation and symptoms like arthritis

- Relieving headaches and other pains (as a pain reliever)

Ginger Tea

Yields 1 Serving

Ingredients

1 or 2 slices of ginger root

Alkaline sweetener of choice (optional)

1 cup boiling water

Directions

Place the slices of ginger root in a mug. Add the boiling water then cover and let it steep for 5-10 minutes. You can also add some agave sugar if desired.

Rosemary

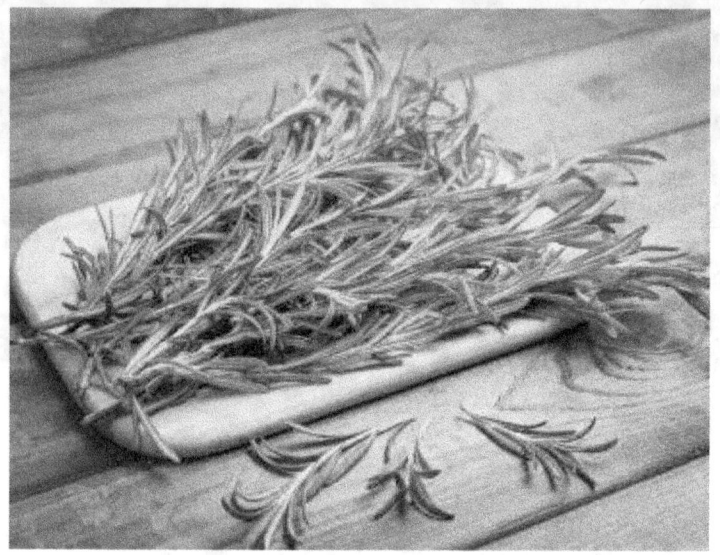

Scientific name: *Rosmarinus officinalis*

Common name: Rosemary

Used parts: leaves, twigs

Common medical uses:

- Boosting the immune system and reducing inflammation

- Improving digestion

- Improving concentration and memory

- Preventing brain aging

- Protecting against muscle degeneration

- Slowing down cancer development

Rosemary Tea

Yields 2 Servings

Ingredients

2-3 teaspoon rosemary leaves/ 1 tablespoon dried rosemary

2 cups water

Directions

Add the rosemary to a cup containing hot water, cover and steep for five or more minutes, depending on how strong you want the tea to be (too long makes it bitter). If you're using fresh rosemary leaves, you can either leave them in as you drink or just strain them out. When using dried leaves, you just have to strain them out before drinking.

Chamomile

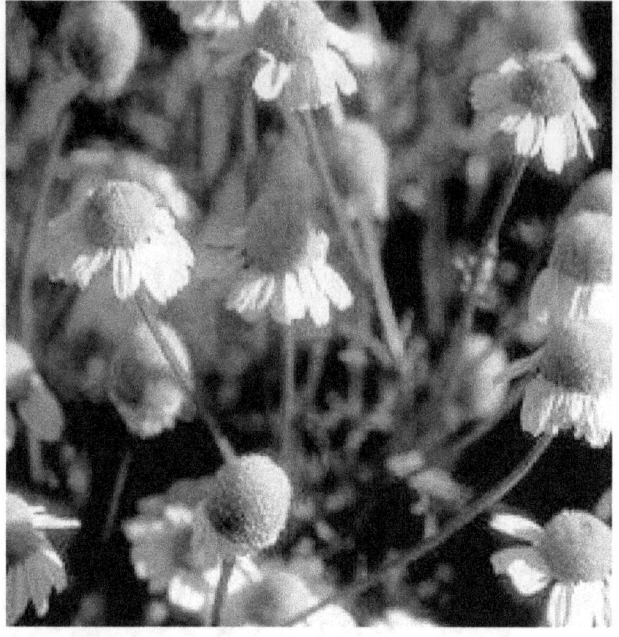

Scientific name: *Matricaria chamomilla*

Common name: Chamomile

Used parts: flowers and leaves

Common medical uses:

- Used as a sedative and antispasmodic in the treatment of rheumatic and digestive disorders

- Treating parasitic worm infections

- Treating ulcers and cleaning wounds

- Promoting granulation and proper healing of the necrotic tissue

- Treating inflammation and bacterial attacks

Chamomile Tea

Yields 2 Servings

Ingredients

2 teaspoon dried chamomile flowers

Sweetener (optional)

2 cups hot water

Directions

Add the boiling water to a cup containing the chamomile flowers and cover. Let them infuse for 2-3 minutes and then strain.

Add a sweetener if you want and serve.

Enjoy!

Green Tea

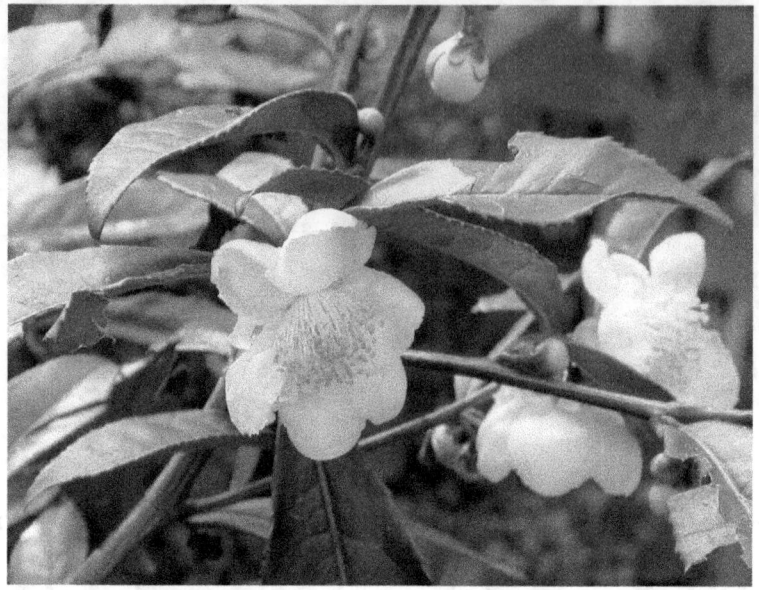

Scientific name: *Camellia sinensis*

Common name: green tea

Used parts: flowers and leaves

Common medical uses:

- Preventing cancer

- Reducing cholesterol

- Preventing or delaying Parkinson's disease

- Treating diarrhea and dysentery

- Treating gastro-enteritis and hepatitis

Green Tea

Yields 1 Serving

Ingredients

Green tea leaves (camellia sinensis)-1 teaspoon for 1 cup of green tea

A tea strainer

1 cup of water

Directions

Measure 1 teaspoon of the green tea leaves if you want to make one cup. You can add more teaspoons if you want to make more tea, but make sure to maintain the ratio.

Now place the leaves in a sieve or strainer and keep aside.

Add the water to a stainless steel pan or pot and bring to a boil. You can also use a glass teapot. The best temperature for green tea is between 80 degrees C. and 85 degrees C. so make sure to keep an eye on the water to ensure it doesn't boil. However, if it starts boiling, just switch the heat off and allow it to cool for a little while- 30-35 seconds is ideal.

Place the strainer or sieve over the mug or cup and then pour the water into the cup then cover. Wait for three minutes, for the tea to steep. You'll need to be careful here though since not everyone likes their tea strong. Therefore, try checking whether the tea is fine. You may want to keep a spoon nearby and drink a spoonful every 30 seconds to see whether the flavor works for you.

Take out the strainer and set aside. You can add a sweetener at this point if you want to.

Olive Leaf

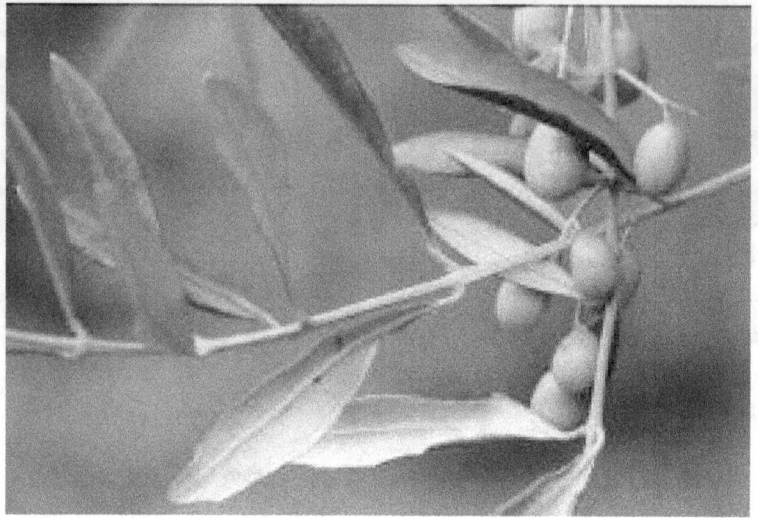

Scientific name: *Olea europaea*

Common name: olive leaf

Used parts: leaves

Common medical uses:

- Treating diabetes

- Improving blood pressure

- Fighting viruses such as rotavirus, herpes and Influenza

- Improving allergies

- Relieving diarrhea

Olive Leaf Tea

Yields 1-2 Servings

Ingredients

20 dried leaves

1 teaspoon of lemon juice (optional)

8 ounces of boiling water

Sweetener

Directions

Add the boiling water to a cup containing the leaves then cover and let it steep for about 10 minutes.

Strain and add a sweetener or lemon if you want, to taste.

Enjoy!

Thyme

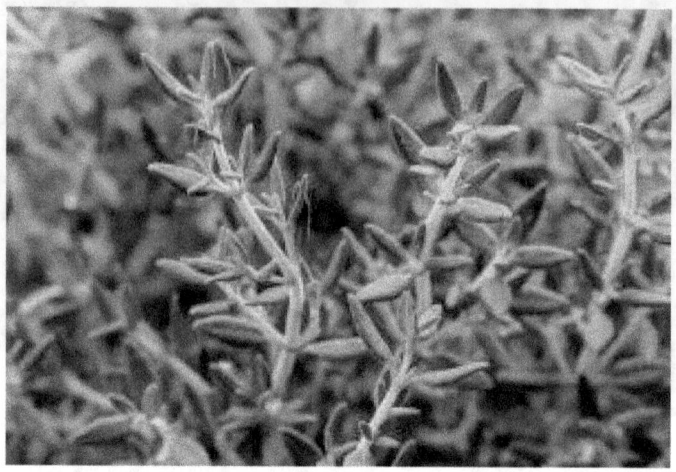

Scientific name: *Thymus vulgaris*

Common name: thyme

Used parts: flowers and leaves

Common medical uses:

- Improving symptoms of breast and colon cancer

- Reducing and treating common skin infections

- Treating yeast infection

- Improving high blood pressure

- Treating arthritis

- Treating diarrhea

Thyme Tea

Yields 1 Serving

Ingredients

1 1/2 cup boiling water

3 sprigs of fresh thyme/ 2 sprigs dried thyme

Directions

Put the thyme springs into a cup and add the boiling water. Cover and give it about five minutes to steep. Remove the sprigs before you drink and enjoy!

Lavender

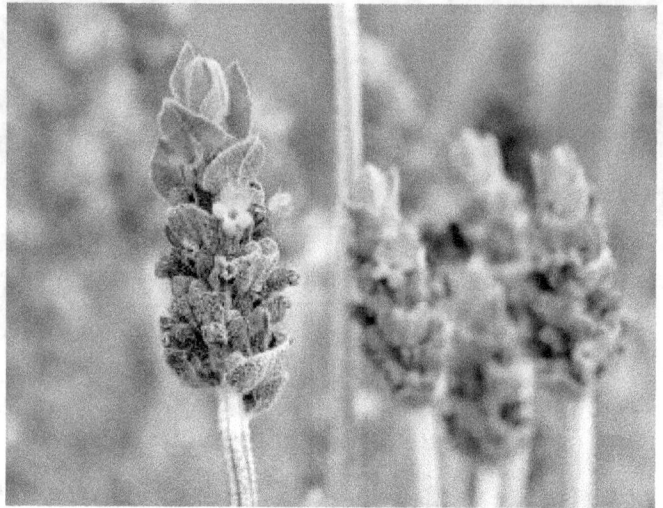

Scientific name: *Lavandula*

Common name: Lavender

Used parts: flowers

Common medical uses:

- Treating anxiety

- Treating fungal infections and wounds

- Treating hair loss

- Stabilizing mood

- Improving sleep

- Soothing the nerves

- Balancing the blood sugar

Lavender Tea

Yields 7 Servings

Ingredients

8 cups boiling water

4 tablespoons culinary lavender buds

Directions

Add the buds to a tea pot and pour the 8 cups of boiling water over them and cover. Give the tea 10 minutes to steep.

Pour the tea into a cup through a strainer.

Add a sweetener as needed.

Sweet Bay

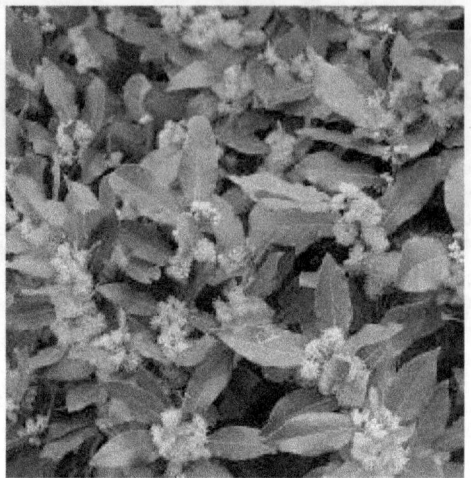

Scientific name: *Laurus nobilis*

Common name: sweet bay

Used parts: leaves and fruit (rarely though)

Common medical uses:

- Treating cancer and gas

- Stimulating the flow of bile

- Triggering sweating

- Treating dandruff

- Relieving pain on the skin, muscle and joints

- Treating boils on the skin

Bay Leaf

Yields 3 Servings

Ingredients

4-5 dried bay leaves

1 liter of water

1 cinnamon stick/ 1 teaspoon ground cinnamon

Directions

Add the bay leaves along with the cinnamon to a cup then add boiling water then cover. Let it steep for 20 or so minutes.

Coriander

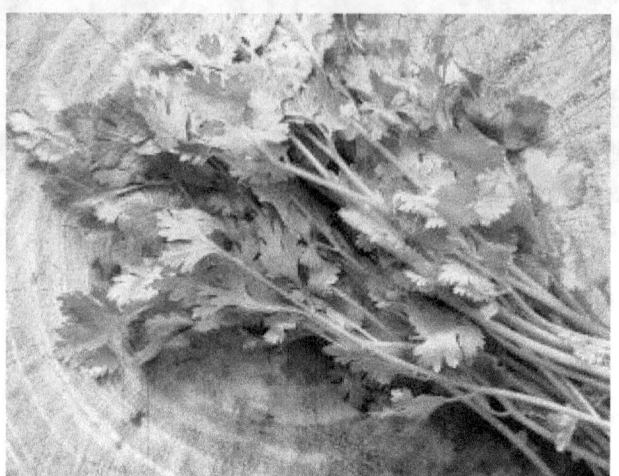

Scientific name: *Coriandrum sativum*

Common name: coriander

Used parts: stems and leaves

Common medical uses:

- Relieving digestion problems, which include diarrhea, stomach upset, intestinal gas and bowel spasms.

- Treating nausea, hernia and loss of appetite

- Treating hemorrhoids and joint pain

- Treating infections caused by fungus and bacteria

- Increasing milk flow in breast-feeding women

- Preventing food poisoning

Coriander Tea

Yields 2 Servings

Ingredients

1/2 teaspoon dried fennel seeds

1/4 teaspoon dried cumin seeds

1/2 teaspoon of dried coriander seeds

Sweetener (optional)

3 cups water

Directions

Grind the coriander seeds in a coffee grinder or spice grinder until they turn to powder.

Boil the water then add it into a container containing the powder and cover. Let it steep for five minutes.

Strain and serve. You can add a sweetener if desired.

Lemon Grass

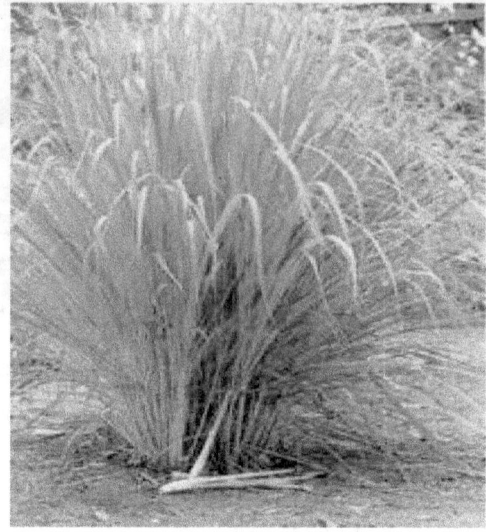

Scientific name: *Cymbopogon citratus*

Common name: lemongrass

Used parts: stems and leaf buds

Common medical uses:

- Reducing anxiety

- Reducing cholesterol

- Preventing fungal infection, especially in people with low immunity

- Reducing inflammation

- Boosting oral health

- Relieving pain

- Boosting the red blood cells

Fresh Lemongrass Tea

Yields 2 Servings

Ingredients

2-3 stalks lemongrass fresh/ dried lemongrass

Black tea bags, to serve (optional)

3 cups water

Lemon slice optional, to serve

Sweetener (optional)

Directions

Add the water to a pot and bring to a boil. If you're using fresh lemongrass, wash and cut it into smaller pieces using a scissor. Pour the boiling water into a container that has all the other ingredients then cover. Let it steep for about ten minutes.

When done, take the tea out of the heat and strain.

Serve immediately, with a slice of lemon, and a sweetener if you want.

Enjoy!

Parsley

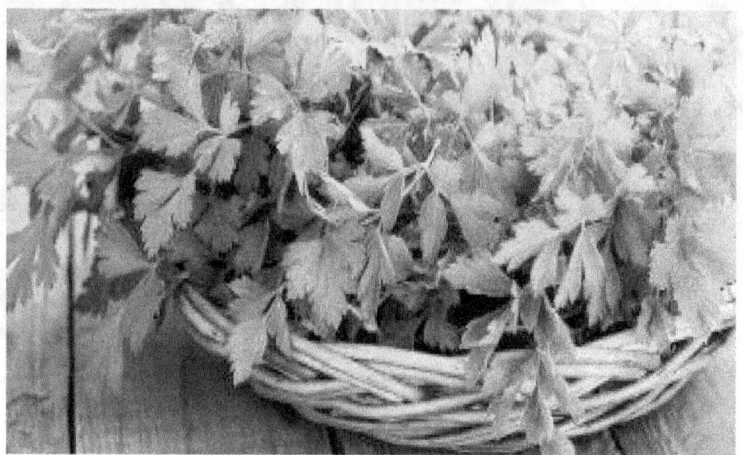

Scientific name: *Petroselinum crispum*

Common name: parsley

Used parts: roots, seeds and leaves

Common medical uses:

- Treating urinary tract infections and gastrointestinal infections

- Preventing constipation

- Improving diabetes, asthma, hypertension and cough

- Improving the skin (removing the cracks, insect bites, bruises and tumors).

- Stimulating hair growth

Parsley Tea

Yields 2 Servings

Ingredients

3 tablespoons dried parsley

A large piece of fresh ginger root

1/2 lemon

Optional sweetener such as agave nectar

Enough water for 2 cups

Directions

Add the water to a kettle and bring to a boil.

Add about two teaspoons of the lemon zest and squeeze the juice from the lemon into a container that can accommodate 2 cups. Then grate one tablespoon of the ginger root and add it into the container with lemons. Add in dried parsley leaves.

Pour the boiling water into the container, stir well and cover then let it steep for 5-7 minutes to steep.

Lastly, strain the juice into your cup and add in a sweetener (if using) while stirring.

Oregano

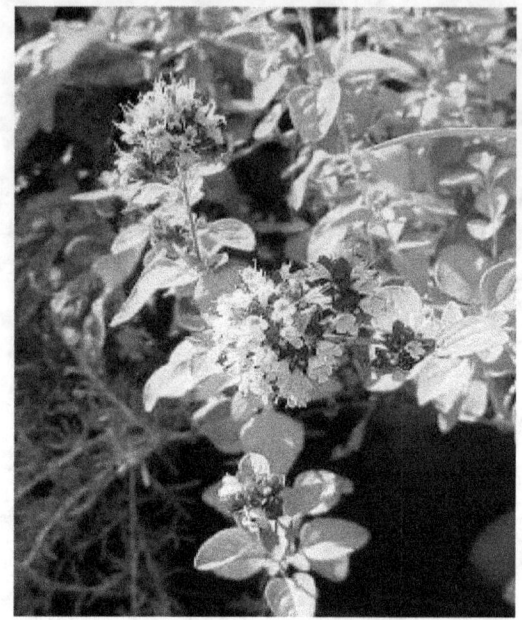

Scientific name: *Origanum vulgare*

Common name: oregano

Used parts: leaves

Common medical uses:

- Treats arthritis

- Relieves colds and flu

- Relieves fatigue

- Relieves migraines

- Relieves sinusitis

- Relieves sore throat

Oregano Tea

Yields 4 Cups

Ingredients

4 cups water

2 tablespoons dried oregano

Agave sugar

Directions

Bring the water to a boil then add the boiling water to a container that has the dried oregano leaves (it should be able to fit 4 cups) and cover. Let it steep for ten minutes.

Pour it into the cups through a strainer.

Serve it immediately. If desired, sweeten the tea with any alkaline sweetener.

NOTE:

In the next book I am working on, you will learn more about herbal medicine. The book will be very detailed on the uses of these and more medicinal plants in curing diseases and maintaining the right physical and mental health.

Conclusion

We have come to the end of the book. Thank you for reading and congratulations for reading until the end.

There you have it! -All the information you need about the alkaline diet, and the breakfast, lunch, dinner and snack recipes you need to get you started and adapted to an alkaline lifestyle. As you can see, following the alkaline diet does not only limit you to certain kinds of food, as there's a wide variety of foods to enjoy.

However, you need to note that the alkaline diet does not mean you go cold turkey on all the foods you like. If they're not alkaline, you can reduce them gradually by combining them with the healthy, alkaline options in each meal, but having smaller and smaller bits of them with every meal until they're completely eliminated. The recipes in this book will help you with this for the simple reason that they are delicious and highly likely to give you an interesting food adventure!

Also, ensure you consume the drinks mentioned in this book (including the ones in the last chapter) after meals to ensure you completely reverse the acidic effects of the foods you're trying to eliminate and make the process easier for your body.

Thank you for staying with me to this point; now you take it from here!

If you found the book valuable, can you recommend it to others? One way to do that is to post a review on Amazon.

Thank you and good luck!

References

Adam E. Ziemann, J. E. (2009). The Amygdala Is a Chemosensor that Detects Carbon Dioxide and Acidosis to Elicit Fear Behavior. *Cell*.

ANNA CHALLA, W. C. (1993). Effect of metabolic acidosis on the expression of insulin-likegrowth factor and growth hormone receptor. *Kidney International*.

Bailey, J. L. (2000). ACID-BASE IN RENAL FAILURE: Twice-Told Tales of Metabolic Acidosis, Glucocorticoids, and Protein Wasting: What Do Results from Rats Tell Us About Patients with Kidney Disease?. *Seminars in Dialysis*.

Buehlmeier, J. R.-M.-G. (2016). Glucocorticoid activity and metabolism with NaCl-induced low-grade metabolic acidosis and oral alkalization: results of two randomized controlled trials. *Endocrine*.

Dawson-Hughes, B. H. (2008). Alkaline diets favor lean tissue mass in older adults. *The American journal of clinical nutrition*.

Despa, F. D. (2013). Amylin: what might be its role in Alzheimer's disease and how could this affect therapy? *Expert review of proteomics*.

Hamm, L. L. (1999). Role of glucocorticoids in acidosis. *American Journal of Kidney Diseases*.

Keiichi Morishita M.D., H. A. (1976). *Hidden Truth of Cancer*. George Ohsawa Macrobiotic Foundation.

Levitan EB, C. N. (2008). Dietary glycemic index, dietary glycemic load, blood lipids, and C-reactive protein. *Metabolism*.

Maurizi, G. D. (2018). Adipocytes properties and crosstalk with immune system in obesity-related inflammation. *Cell Physiol*.

McCarty, M. (2000). *The origins of western obesity: a role for animal protein? - PubMed - NCBI.*

McMillan-Price J, P. P. (2006). Comparison of 4 Diets of Varying Glycemic Load on Weight Loss and Cardiovascular Risk Reduction in Overweight and Obese Young Adults: A Randomized Controlled Trial. *Arch Intern Med.*

PEDERSEN, S. B. (1996). Identification of steroid receptors in human adipose tissue. *European Journal of Clinical Investigation.*

Rebuffé-Scrive, M. B.-A. (1990). Steroid Hormone Receptors in Human Adipose Tissues. *The Journal of Clinical Endocrinology & Metabolism.*

Robey, I. F. (2012). Examining the relationship between diet-induced acidosis and cancer. *Nutrition & Metabolism.*

Schwalfenberg, G. K. (2012). The Alkaline Diet: Is There Evidence That an Alkaline pH Diet Benefits Health? *Journal of Environmental and Public Health.*

Schwalfenberg, G. K. (2012). The Alkaline Diet: Is There Evidence That an Alkaline pH Diet Benefits Health? *Journal of Environmental and Public Health.*

Scott, R. B. (2018). Problem or solution: The strange story of glucagon. *Peptides.*

Stanhope, K. L. (2016). Sugar consumption, metabolic disease and obesity: The state of the controversy. *Critical Reviews in Clinical Laboratory Sciences.*

Stanhope, K. L. (2016). Sugar consumption, metabolic disease and obesity: The state of the controversy. *Critical Reviews in Clinical Laboratory Sciences.*

Vos, M. B. (2008). Dietary Fructose Consumption Among US Children and Adults: The Third National Health and Nutrition Examination Survey. *The Medscape Journal of Medicine.*

Williams, R. S.-B. (2016). Dietary acid load, metabolic acidosis and insulin resistance - Lessons from cross-sectional and overfeeding studies in humans. *Clinical Nutrition (Edinburgh, Scotland)* .

Williams, R. S.-B. (2016, May). The role of dietary acid load and mild metabolic acidosis in insulin resistance in humans. *Biochimie.*